SOMATIC EXERCISES

FOR BEGINNERS BOOK

Simple Exercises For Nervous System Regulation, Releasing Trauma, Reducing Tension, and Alleviate Pain and Stress.

Luna Light

Contents

HEAD, NECK, AND SHOULDERS RELEASE

BACK RELEASE

LOWER BODY RELEASE

FOOT EXERCISES

COMBINATION MOVEMENTS

What This Book Can Do For You

"Through the body, we realize we are a spark of divinity."
– Ida Rolf. Creator of Rolfing

Congratulations!

Why am I congratulating you?

Because you just made a purchase that can truly transform your body if you put it into action. There are a lot of "Somatic exercise" books on Amazon, and you made the right decision picking this one. Here's why:

Unlike my competitors who are business people with no knowledge of Somatic work, I am actually someone whose life was saved by Somatic movements. I survived a near-fatal car accident and only through these movements did I regain my strength and overcome chronic pain and was finally able to walk again. I owe my life to the work of Thomas Hanna, the founder of Somatic movements.

All the other "Somatic exercise" books are published by entrepreneurs gaming the Amazon ranking system to make money. They repurpose "Somatic exercises" by slightly altering normal yoga or Pilates stretches, but these are not the true Somatic movements.

A real Somatic movement, as taught to me by Thomas Hanna and his wife Eleanor Criswell Hanna at her clinic in Sonoma, uses pandiculation to relax tense muscles and restore their natural calm state. You will learn what pandiculation is in this book, and how to incorporate it into smooth, calming movements so you can restore your body's strength and its natural flow state.

P.S. If you want to get straight to the exercises, please go to page 41.

Let's get into it!

Love,

-Luna Light

The Origins of Somatic Exercises

Derived from the Greek word *soma*, which means "the living body," Somatic practices are rooted in the understanding that our bodies are repositories of emotions and experiences.

The essence of Somatic exercises lies in their ability to foster a re-engagement and reintegration of the body and mind. Through gentle movements, focused attention, and conscious breathing, these exercises enable individuals to explore and alter their physiological responses of stress and trauma.

Historically, cultures around the world have always recognized the significance of the body in emotional and spiritual well-being, employing various forms of dance, touch, and movement as modalities of healing.

In the 20th century, this understanding evolved within the field of psychotherapy with pioneers like Wilhelm Reich, who emphasized the role of the body in manifesting emotional disturbances, and later, practitioners like Moshe Feldenkrais and Alexander Lowen developed techniques that explicitly combined physical and mental health practices. This led to the development of the Feldenkrais Method and the Alexander Method, both of which have produced many teachers even to this day.

Today, when mental and physical ailments are often treated with quick fixes or suppressive medications, Somatic exercises offer a different path. They provide a method for individuals to slowly unravel the layers of tension, resistance, and disconnection that accumulate over a lifetime.

For those suffering from conditions like anxiety, depression, PTSD, and physical ailments such as chronic pain, Somatic exercises offer a way to deeply understand and renegotiate their relationship with their bodies.[1]

When all the MRIs, blood tests and health checkups are done and you still sense your body is weak or somehow under stress, Somatic exercises are a good place to continue your search. If you are able to find some other medical issue, most of the time, the gentle Somatic movements can supplement your recovery with slow, controlled trauma release of emotions and physical stress in your body.

---

1   It's important to rule out physical or other medical and psychological causes first before coming to this conclusion. However it can be done in conjunction with other forms of medical treatments.

Overview of Somatic Exercises

This book will introduce a variety of Somatic exercises, each tailored to facilitate a specific aspect of your body. These exercises range from simple practices like mindful breathing and slow, deliberate movements to more complex sequences that require attention to the body's responses and the emotions they evoke.

You may feel different emotions or memories come up as you progress through these movements. Don't worry, this is normal. It's just trauma leaving the body. If a particular emotion or memory seems too much at the moment, go back to laying on the ground or any comfortable position for you and take a few breathes. Feel free to pause or stop at any time if you feel discomfort or need a break.

As you engage with these exercises, you will be invited to notice the sensations, no matter how subtle, and to explore the messages these sensations convey about your emotional and physical state. This process of attentive engagement is crucial as it fosters a deeper ability to sense and process your emotions. This is critical for letting trapped emotions go.

In short, this book will help you start to hear the stories your body has been wanting to tell, heal the wounds you carry, and take back the joy and vitality that are naturally yours.

Before we dive into the exercises, let's quickly explore the founder of Somatic movements, Thomas Hannah.

The Founder of Somatic Movements: Thomas Hanna

In his seminal book, *Bodies in Revolt: A Primer in Somatic Thinking* in 1970, Thomas Hanna introduced a profound shift from traditional exercise paradigms towards a more integrated and aware engagement with our bodily selves.

Hanna saw the human body not just as a mechanical system but as a holistic combination of your emotions, energy frequency and mechanics.

I could bore you with all of Thomas Hanna's accomplishments, but the short version is that Hanna was a well-studied professor at the University of Florida who transitioned into the Humanistic Psychology Institute in San Francisco, beginning his work in developing the field of Somatics.

The essence of Somatics, as Hanna conceived it, is rooted in the Greek word "soma," meaning the living body in its wholeness. Unlike conventional exercises, which often emphasize repetition and external form, Somatics focuses on the internal experience of movement. It encourages heightened sensory awareness and the mindful correction of physical patterns that cause pain or limitation.

Hanna's methods, particularly his development of Clinical Somatic Education, diverge from traditional approaches by emphasizing self-awareness and internal control over muscles through a process he described as "sensory-motor education." This process allows individuals to retrain their bodies to overcome sensory-motor amnesia: the loss of control over certain muscle groups which results in chronic pain, tension and decreased flexibility as we age.

In his sessions, which attracted clients worldwide, Hanna utilized gentle, explorative movements that helped individuals rediscover their natural ability to move freely. This approach not only addressed specific physical ailments but also improved overall well-being, embodying Hanna's belief that "freedom of the body reflects freedom of the spirit."

In his first Somatic movements book, Hanna described seeing Moshe Feldenkrais as a young professor working on a man whose body was so twisted he had trouble walking. The man walked up to the table on the stage and Feldenkrais proceeded to work on him for 15 min. After the session, the man looked up, and suddenly began to move and walk around. Moshe enjoyed doing these demonstrations in lectures, and when Hanna saw the results, he was hooked. This was the spark that led him to developing a completely new method of understanding the body that diverged from the Alexander Technique and the Feldenkrais Method.

Somatics, under Hanna's guidance, developed a unique language and methodology for understanding the body's pain and responses as not merely physiological but deeply tied to emotional states and life histories. His movements focused on reversing the stretch response to focus on pandiculation, the releasing of tense muscles. We'll show you how this works using the exercises in this book.

The impact of Thomas Hanna's work extends beyond his books and teachings at the Somatic Systems Institute. Somatics has influenced various fields of therapy, physical health, and personal development, offering a holistic approach to healing that acknowledges the body's role as an integral part of the psycho-emotional self.

What is Pandiculation?

The main pillar of the Somatic exercises is **Pandiculation**.

Pandiculation is a term that might not be widely recognized outside certain scientific and therapeutic communities, yet it represents a fundamental, instinctual practice observed throughout the animal kingdom. You might notice it when a cat yawns or a dog performs the downward dog stretch after waking up.

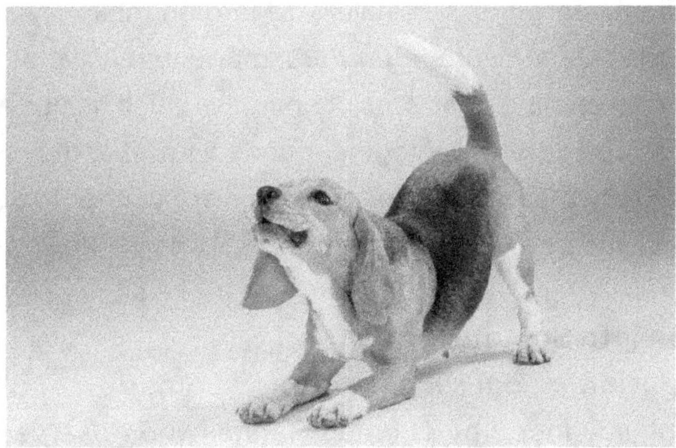

This natural process, which involves the stretching and tensing of the muscles followed by their complete relaxation, is something we subconsciously engage in, particularly when yawning upon waking or after long periods of inactivity.

At its core, pandiculation is the act of stretching and contracting the muscles in a coordinated, yawn-like fashion, which is then followed by relaxation. This action is not only a stretch but a voluntary, controlled contraction of muscles throughout the body. It is a holistic, reflexive maneuver that helps to reset the muscle tone by regulating the tension level and preparing it for efficient movement.

Historical Background

The concept of pandiculation can be traced back to the natural behavior observed in animals, particularly mammals, which often perform this action upon waking. The etymology of the word itself, stemming from the Latin *pandiculari*, which means "to stretch oneself," hints at this deeply ingrained physical routine. Despite its ubiquitous nature, pandiculation has only been studied in depth in more recent times, especially within the context of modern Somatic practices and its applications in therapeutic settings.

Early Observations

Pandiculation was observed and noted by naturalists and biologists who studied animal behaviors, particularly regarding their rest and activity cycles. Charles Darwin, among others, made extensive notes on the yawning and stretching behaviors of animals, which he correlated with emotional states and physiological needs. However, it was not until the 20th century that these observations were connected to broader physiological and psychological theories.

Integration into Somatic Education

The integration of pandiculation into Somatic education was significantly advanced by Thomas Hanna, who observed that this natural act could have profound implications for human health and mobility.

In his development of Clinical Somatic Education, Hanna recognized pandiculation as a key component in retraining the nervous system to release chronic muscle tension.

By deliberately contracting and then slowly releasing muscles, individuals could relearn how to control their muscle states and reduce the effects of involuntary, chronic muscular contraction that often leads to pain and reduced mobility.

How Pandiculation Works

Pandiculation is a simple yet profound technique that works in three key stages to help your muscles relax more deeply than traditional stretching. Let's break down each stage:

1. **Voluntary Muscle Contraction**: The first step is to voluntarily contract the muscle you're focusing on, making it slightly tighter than its current state. This intentional tightening is crucial because it sends a clear signal to your brain, pinpointing the exact muscles that need attention. This contraction is about providing your brain with precise information on where to direct its efforts.

2. **Slow Controlled Release:** After the contraction, the next step is to slowly release the muscle. This isn't just about letting go; it's about carefully controlling the muscle's return to a relaxed state. This slow release allows your brain to recalibrate the muscle's length and tension according to the new data it has received. It's during this phase that your brain effectively regains control over the muscle, adjusting it to operate optimally.

3. **Complete Relaxation:** The final stage is complete relaxation. Once the muscle has been slowly released, allowing it to fully relax helps the brain to integrate this new state of muscle function. This integration is vital as it helps cement the muscle's new settings, preventing the old patterns of excessive tightness from immediately returning.

The Science of Pandiculation

The physiological basis of pandiculation lies in its ability to reset the muscle length and tension set points at the level of the nervous system. When muscles contract, they send sensory feedback to the brain about their state and length. By intentionally tightening and then slowly relaxing the muscles, pandiculation provides the nervous system with a fresh set of data on the state of the muscles, effectively resetting the muscle length and tension to a more optimal state.

Neurological Effects

From a neurological perspective, pandiculation stimulates the alpha motor neurons, which are responsible for muscle contraction, and the sensory receptors within the muscles, known as muscle spindles. This stimulation helps to recalibrate the communication between the muscles and the central nervous system, enhancing proprioception—the body's sense of its own position in space—and muscular control.

Therapeutic Benefits

Clinically, pandiculation has been incorporated into various therapeutic practices to help treat conditions related to muscle tension and rigidity, such as chronic back pain, stiffness associated with conditions like Parkinson's disease and general muscular fatigue. It is particularly valued in fields like physical therapy, yoga, and other movement therapies for its efficacy in improving flexibility, reducing muscular pain, and enhancing overall physical responsiveness.

Pandiculation in Animals

Animals, especially mammals, exhibit pandiculation frequently—most notably upon waking from sleep. This behavior is not just a random stretch; it is a coordinated sequence of actions that involves extending the limbs and arching the back and is often accompanied by a wide opening of the mouth in a yawn. The purpose of this action goes beyond simple stretching; it serves to awaken the nervous system, re-oxygenate the blood, and reset the muscle fibers after periods of inactivity.

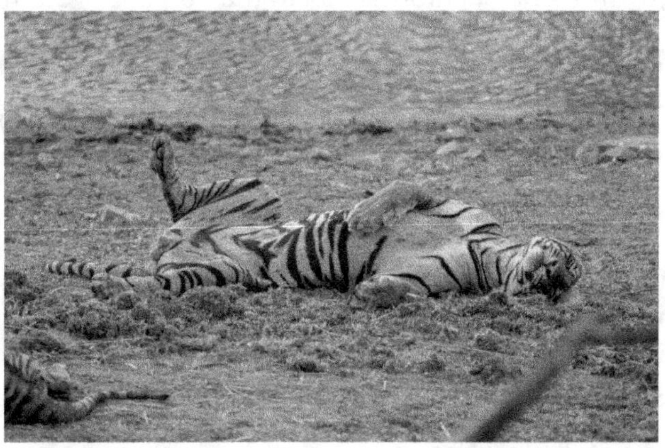

Zoologists and animal behaviorists suggest that pandiculation is crucial for survival in the wild, as it prepares an animal's body for the demands of immediate physical activity, such as fleeing from predators or resuming hunting after rest. For instance, a lion awakening from rest demonstrates pronounced pandiculation, visibly contracting its powerful leg muscles before slowly releasing them. **This action ensures that the muscles are less stiff and more responsive, optimizing the animal's readiness for rapid, explosive movements necessary for chasing down prey.**

In humans, pandiculation is often manifested in the form of stretching and yawning upon waking or after being stationary for extended durations. **It is a natural response to the reduced muscle tone and decreased bodily awareness that comes with sleep or prolonged sitting**. As in animals, this behavior in humans serves multiple physiological and psychological purposes:

1. **Muscle Reawakening:** Pandiculation helps to wake up the muscles by increasing blood flow and stimulating the muscle spindles, which are sensors within the muscles that communicate length and tension information to the nervous system.

2. **Resetting the Nervous System:** By intentionally contracting and then relaxing the muscles, pandiculation helps recalibrate the body's sense of muscle tone and position, which can be altered by periods of inactivity or disuse.

3. **Stress Relief:** Pandiculating also appears to have a psychological component, offering a form of stress relief. The deep stretch and subsequent release can be profoundly satisfying, helping to relieve feelings of tension and contributing to a sense of physical and mental relaxation.

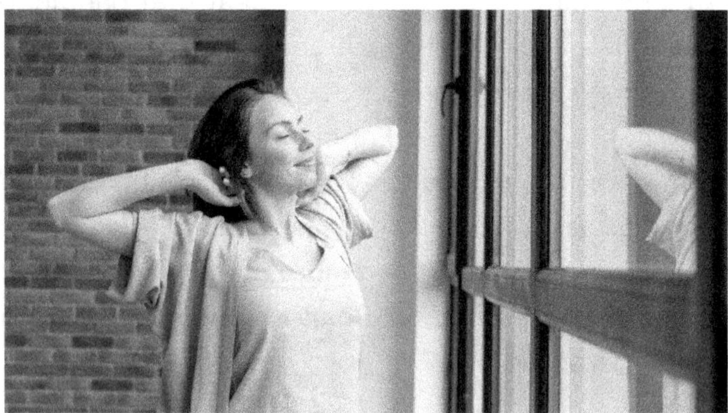

Neurological and Physiological Perspectives

From a neurological perspective, pandiculation is all about improving the brain's control over muscle function. When you pandiculate, you start by contracting a muscle intentionally—this sends a strong signal to your brain about the state of that muscle. Essentially, you're telling your brain, "Hey, look here, pay attention to this area." This is helpful because our brains sometimes lose track of how tense our muscles are, especially if we've been sitting still for a long time or if we're stressed.

After contracting the muscle, you then slowly release it. This slow release is crucial because it allows the brain to process how the muscle is lengthening and becoming more relaxed. It's like updating the brain's map of the body. This updated map helps the brain know exactly how the muscle feels when it's relaxed versus when it's tense.

Finally, complete relaxation helps solidify this new information in the brain. It's a chance for the brain to "save" this updated status, much like saving a document on your computer. This step is essential for making lasting changes to how the muscles feel and function.

Physiologically, pandiculation affects more than just muscle tension. It can influence how blood flows through your muscles, how nerves communicate pain, and overall how relaxed or energetic you feel. Regularly practicing pandiculation can lead to better muscle coordination, reduced muscle fatigue, and even decreased pain. This is particularly important for people who may have chronic pain or stiffness due to conditions like arthritis or repetitive strain injuries.

Moreover, pandiculation doesn't just help with physical aspects; it has a calming effect on the mind too. The act of focusing on moving and relaxing muscles can be meditative, helping to reduce stress and anxiety.

Pandiculation vs. Traditional Stretching

Pandiculation is an instinctive, physiological process involving the deliberate tightening or contracting of muscles followed by a slow, controlled release. This action, often accompanied by yawning, is not just about stretching the muscles but about resetting the muscle length and tone through the central nervous system. It's a neuromuscular re-education of sorts, teaching the body to release chronic tension and improve muscular control.

Traditional stretching, on the other hand, typically involves holding a pose that elongates specific muscles or muscle groups to increase range of motion and flexibility. This form of stretching is passive compared to the active engagement of muscles in pandiculation. The focus is primarily on the mechanical aspects of increasing muscle length and elasticity without necessarily engaging the nervous system in the same recalibration process.

Mechanisms and Effects

- **Neuromuscular Resetting:** Pandiculation acts directly on the nervous system. By consciously contracting and then slowly releasing muscles, it provides the brain with feedback about the state of muscle tension and length. This process helps to reset the gamma loop, which is responsible for adjusting the sensitivity of muscle spindles, crucial for proper muscle function. The result is a natural adjustment of muscle tone, potentially reducing the likelihood of muscle injuries and chronic tension.

- **Flexibility and Range of Motion:** Traditional stretching impacts flexibility by mechanically lengthening the muscle fibers, which can help improve overall range of motion and decrease the risk of injuries during physical activities. While effective in promoting elasticity, traditional stretches do not engage the nervous system in a manner that leads to neuromuscular reeducation or a resetting of muscle tone.

Benefits and Limitations

Benefits of Pandiculation:

- **Engages the Whole Body:** Pandiculation involves a holistic approach, affecting the muscular, nervous, and even lymphatic systems, facilitating a comprehensive body awakening and reconditioning.

- **Reduces Muscle Tension:** By resetting muscle tone, pandiculation can alleviate the discomfort of chronic muscular tension and stiffness, often more effectively than traditional stretching.

- **Improves Proprioception:** The active engagement required in pandiculation enhances body awareness, or proprioception, which is crucial for balance and coordinated movement.

Benefits of Traditional Stretching:

- **Increases Flexibility:** Regular stretching can lead to significant improvements in flexibility, which is beneficial for both daily activities and athletic performance.

- **Promotes Relaxation:** Static stretching can help relax muscles and is often used as part of cooldown routines to help the body transition to a restful state after exercise.

Limitations of Each Approach:

- **Pandiculation** requires a level of conscious engagement and understanding of one's body signals, which might be challenging for some, especially without proper guidance.

- While beneficial, **traditional stretching** can sometimes lead to overstretching or injuries if not performed correctly, and it lacks the neuromuscular component that pandiculation provides.

Neuromuscular Reeducation through Pandiculation

One of the key distinctions of active pandiculation is its ability to reset the sensory-motor system. By contracting the muscles before stretching, pandiculation stimulates the muscle spindles: sensory receptors that inform the brain about muscle length and tension.

This intentional engagement followed by a deliberate release helps recalibrate the body's proprioceptive map, which is essential for coordinating movement and maintaining posture.

For individuals experiencing chronic pain, trauma, or bodily stress, this reeducation of the nervous system can lead to profound shifts in how they experience and inhabit their bodies.

Psychological and Physiological Impacts

The psychological impacts of active pandiculation are significant and align closely with trauma recovery processes. Pandiculation allows individuals to actively participate in their healing process, offering a sense of control and agency that is often compromised in trauma survivors.

By engaging in a conscious dialogue with their bodies through pandiculation, individuals can gently explore the edges of their physical capacity, often expanding their range of motion and reducing the hyper arousal of the nervous system.

Conversely, passive stretching, while less engaging, provides a low-demand method to maintain muscle elasticity and joint mobility. It can be particularly beneficial in settings where active engagement might be too challenging or intense, providing a gentle approach to maintaining physical health.

Integration in Therapeutic Practices

For therapists and practitioners working within the Somatic and psychological frameworks, integrating pandiculation into treatment plans can enhance outcomes for those dealing with Somatic symptoms of stress and trauma. It offers a hands-on approach that empowers individuals to reconnect with their bodies in a safe and controlled manner.

Central Nervous System is the command center

The central nervous system (CNS), which comprises the brain and spinal cord, is at the core of muscle control and relaxation. The CNS functions as the command center, sending and receiving signals that govern muscle movement and relaxation. This intricate system coordinates voluntary movements and involuntary responses, regulating everything from deliberate actions like walking to reflexive reactions like flinching.

Motor Neurons act as the messengers

Motor neurons play a crucial role in muscle control. Originating in the brainstem and spinal cord, these neurons send impulses that pass through the nervous system to the muscles, instructing them to contract or relax. The efficiency and health of these neurons are essential for smooth, coordinated muscle movements. In conditions where the motor neurons are disrupted—such as in certain neurological disorders—the resulting muscle control can be markedly impaired, manifesting as spasticity or muscle weakness.

Autonomic Nervous System:

Parallel to the CNS, the autonomic nervous system (ANS) operates largely outside of conscious control, managing the body's automatic functions like heart rate, digestion, and, yes, muscle relaxation. The ANS is split into two main branches:

- **The Sympathetic Nervous System**, often described as the 'fight or flight' system, prepares the body for acute stress by increasing the heart rate, expanding the airways, and tensing the muscles.

- **The Parasympathetic Nervous System**, or the 'rest and digest' system, counters this activation, calming the body by slowing the heart rate, constricting the airways, and facilitating muscle relaxation.

Balancing Act

In the context of trauma, the balance between these two systems can become skewed, with the sympathetic nervous system remaining in a constant state of alert, often leading to chronic muscle tension: a common complaint among those with PTSD. Herein lies the critical role of Somatic exercises, which can engage the parasympathetic nervous system and help restore balance, promoting relaxation and healing.

Neuroplasticity:

A key concept in understanding how Somatic exercises can affect muscle control and relaxation is neuroplasticity—the brain's ability to reorganize itself by forming new neural connections throughout life.

This ability is crucial for recovery from trauma and stress disorders, as it allows the brain to adapt to new experiences and environments. By engaging in practices that promote relaxation and mindful muscle control, individuals can essentially 'rewire' their brains, diminishing maladaptive neural pathways and strengthening those that support health and well-being.

Engaging the Brain and Nervous System

Somatic exercises specifically target these neural mechanisms. By focusing on mindful movement and awareness of bodily sensations, these exercises encourage a heightened state of proprioception; awareness of the body in space, which is regulated by the CNS. This not only aids in muscle control but also in calibrating the nervous system's response to stress and relaxation.

Moreover, these exercises often incorporate techniques that activate the vagus nerve, a crucial part of the parasympathetic nervous system.

Stimulation of the vagus nerve through deep breathing, gentle stretching, and relaxation techniques can enhance parasympathetic activity, promoting a state of calm and reducing muscle tension.

Sensory Motor Amnesia (SMA): What Happens As We Age

Throughout our lives, our bodies undergo various forms of stress, physical injuries, emotional upheavals, and the inevitable aging process. Each of these factors can leave a lasting imprint on our physical selves, particularly on how we control and experience our muscular functions.

One phenomenon that vividly illustrates this impact is Sensory Motor Amnesia (SMA), a condition I've observed and studied extensively in the context of trauma recovery and body awareness.

Sensory Motor Amnesia encapsulates the idea that our bodies, besieged by the accumulations of life's stressors, can forget how to function optimally, losing the innate fluidity and ease of movements once taken for granted.

What Is Sensory Motor Amnesia

At its core, Sensory Motor Amnesia is a condition in which the brain loses its ability to fully control and sense the muscles. This isn't a problem of muscle mechanics alone; rather, it's a disruption in the neurological communication between the brain and the body.

"Sensory" refers to sensing or feeling, "motor" denotes movement, and "amnesia" means forgetting. Thus, Sensory Motor Amnesia literally means forgetting how to sense and move your muscles effectively.

This forgetfulness isn't about the loss of memory you might associate with names or faces; it's a more insidious type of forgetting, one that creeps into our physical habits. Over time, due to various stresses such as accidents, injuries, surgeries, repetitive stress, or emotional traumas, our muscles learn to stay tight.

This chronic tension can manifest as persistent back pain, neck or shoulder discomfort, or a general sense of bodily imbalance—all signs that the body has adapted to stress in a way that is no longer healthy or sustainable.

The Process of Muscle Retention

Why does this happen? The answer lies in the brain's remarkable ability to adapt. When faced with stress, the body's initial reactions—tightening of muscles, heightened alertness, and increased heart rate, are all protective and adaptive in the short term.

However, when these reactions persist long past the original stressor, they become maladaptive. The brain, operating on outdated data, continues to send signals to the muscles to remain in a state of alert, leading to the rigidity and discomfort characteristic of SMA.

SMA As We Age

As we age, the stakes become higher. Our bodies naturally lose some flexibility and strength, and the presence of Sensory Motor Amnesia can exacerbate these changes, making us more prone to injuries and reducing our quality of life.

The muscles, having learned to lock in patterns of tension, may contribute to a progressive decline in mobility that many accept as a normal part of aging.

However, it's crucial to understand that while some changes in muscle and joint function are inevitable, many aspects of our diminished physical capacity are not only due to aging but to untreated SMA.

Reversing Sensory Motor Amnesia

The good news is that because SMA is a learned response, it can be unlearned. This is where Somatic exercises come into play. These exercises, central to the practice I advocate, are designed not only to stretch or strengthen muscles but to reeducate the brain and body about movement and sensation.

Through gentle, conscious movements that reawaken the brain's control of muscles and movement, Somatic exercises help to release ingrained muscular patterns.

This reeducation process involves slow, mindful movements that allow the brain to 'relearn' the full range of muscle motion. By consciously moving in ways that counteract the habitual patterns, you can gradually restore muscle function and reduce the effects of SMA. This is not an overnight fix but a gentle path to reclaiming the body's capabilities.

Embracing a New Paradigm of Aging

Addressing Sensory Motor Amnesia through Somatic exercises allows us to challenge the conventional wisdom about aging. It allows us to view our older years as an opportunity for regeneration and improved body awareness rather than a period of inevitable decline.

By maintaining an ongoing dialogue through Somatics between the brain and the body, we can continue to move with freedom, balance, and ease, reducing pain and enhancing our overall well-being as we age. For a good example of this, search for one of my teachers on YouTube "Essential Somatics" or "Martha Peterson Somatics". She's in her 70s and still moves like a 20-something!

The Conflict Within Static Stretching

Many of us have been taught the value of static stretching for improving flexibility and reducing muscle tension. However, the underlying mechanics of the stretch reflex can make static stretching less effective than anticipated.

During static stretching, there is an inherent conflict between the voluntary effort to stretch and the involuntary stretch reflex that seeks to contract and protect the muscle. This battle can limit the effectiveness of stretching in achieving lasting changes in muscle tension.

The Temporary Nature of Stretching Benefits

When static stretching is performed, several temporary changes can make us feel more flexible. Initially, if a stretch is held for a prolonged period, the muscle spindles adapt to the new length, reducing their activity and allowing the muscle to remain elongated for a short while. This temporary reduction in spindle sensitivity is why we may feel looser immediately following a stretch.

However, this sensation is fleeting. The stretch reflex gradually returns to its normal vigilance, often within a few hours, leading to the re-tightening of muscles. This cyclical nature of stretching and re-tightening can create a perceived need to stretch frequently, though it does not provide a lasting solution to muscle tension.

Building Tolerance to Stretching

Another aspect of repeated stretching is the development of a tolerance to the sensation of pulling in the muscles. Over time, what may initially feel uncomfortable can become more tolerable, even pleasurable, as the body adapts to the sensation. This adaptation can lead to a sort of dependency on stretching, driven by the temporary relief it provides, rather than any long-term improvements in muscle function or health.

A Better Approach: Pandiculation

To truly address muscle tension and enhance flexibility in a way that aligns with our body's natural mechanisms, we turn to pandiculation.

This technique involves consciously contracting and then slowly releasing the muscles, an action that engages both the muscle spindles and the nervous system in a way that resets muscle tone more effectively than passive stretching.

Pandiculation allows for a re-education of the muscular system, teaching the brain and body to regain control over muscle length and tension without triggering the protective contraction typical of the stretch reflex.

This method provides a sustainable path to improved muscle function, enhanced flexibility, and overall well-being, proving to be a far more effective approach than static stretching for long-term health.

Setting Up Your Safe Space

The space in which we engage in these exercises plays a crucial role in the effectiveness of each session. It should foster a sense of safety, comfort, and tranquility, allowing the mind to focus fully on the body's sensations without external distractions.

The first step in preparing for pandiculation exercises is to establish a dedicated space. This doesn't necessarily require an expansive area or a specialized room but should be a designated spot that signals to your brain that entering this space means entering a time of focusing on and connecting with your body. This psychological and physical boundary helps to cultivate a routine and ritual, enhancing the mind-body connection that is central to Somatic experiencing.

Characteristics of a Suitable Space

1. Minimal Distractions

Choose a location where interruptions are minimized. This means considering both auditory and visual distractions. In a home environment, it might be a quiet corner of a bedroom or a peaceful section of a living room that can be temporarily secluded. The goal is to isolate the space from household traffic or noise from streets and neighbors. If necessary, use sound-masking devices such as white noise machines or soft background music that does not draw attention but instead blends into the background, facilitating deeper focus and relaxation.

2. Adequate Space

Ensure that the area provides enough floor space to lie down fully, stretch out your arms and legs, and move freely without constraints. A clear space not only prevents physical accidents but also promotes a psychological sense of freedom and openness. This is particularly important in pandiculation exercises, where the freedom to extend fully and contract is key to engaging effectively with the exercise.

3. Comfortable Flooring

While pandiculation exercises do not typically require vigorous movement, comfort underfoot is important. Using a yoga mat or a thick rug can provide cushioning and warmth, which helps reduce the hardness of the floor and makes it more comfortable to engage in exercises that involve lying down or sitting. Comfort underfoot is crucial as it also helps maintain positions for longer periods without discomfort. This in turn allows for a deeper focus on the neuromuscular engagement and relaxation phases of pandiculation.

4. Appropriate Lighting

Lighting should be soothing and conducive to relaxation. Harsh lighting can be a distraction and inhibit the ability to relax deeply. Soft, ambient lighting not only soothes the eyes but also helps maintain a calm and serene environment that supports internal focus and mindfulness during exercises.

5. Personalization

Adding personal touches to the space can significantly enhance the experience. This might include elements such as plants, which add a touch of nature and life, or inspirational items like artwork or photos that elicit a sense of peace and tranquility. The personalization of the space should resonate with a sense of safety and comfort, making it a welcoming retreat for daily practice.

6. Preparing Yourself for the Session

Before beginning pandiculation exercises, it's beneficial to spend a few moments grounding yourself in the environment you have created. This might involve sitting quietly, focusing on your breath, and consciously releasing the concerns of the day. Such practices help in transitioning from the outward focus of daily life to the inward focus necessary for effective Somatic work.

How to Mentally and Physically Prepare for Somatic Exercises

The body's responses are not only reactions to physical manipulations but are deeply intertwined with our mental states. Here, I'll guide you through the essential steps to mentally and physically prepare for Somatic exercises, facilitating a holistic engagement with this transformative practice.

Enhancing Body Awareness

1. Body Scanning

Before commencing with Somatic exercises, engage in a body scan. This involves mentally scanning your body from head to toe, noticing any areas of tension, discomfort, or ease. This technique not only heightens your awareness of your bodily state but also helps pinpoint areas that may need more focused attention during your exercises.

2. Conscious Breathing

The way we breathe significantly impacts our ability to engage in Somatic exercises effectively. Start by practicing deep, diaphragmatic breathing. Place one hand on your chest and the other on your belly. Breathe deeply through your nose, ensuring that the diaphragm inflates with enough air to create a stretch in the lungs. Exhale slowly and thoughtfully. This type of breathing enhances oxygen exchange, activates the parasympathetic nervous system, and reduces tension and anxiety, setting a calm, receptive state for the body and mind.

3. Synchronization of Breath and Movement

As you begin your Somatic exercises, synchronize your movements with your breath. For instance, initiate a movement on an inhale and relax or expand on an exhale. This synchronization helps in maintaining a rhythmic flow in exercises, ensuring that movements are not rushed and that the body's internal rhythms align with physical actions.

Emotional Readiness

4. Acknowledging Emotional States

It is essential to acknowledge your emotional state before you start your exercises. Somatic exercises can sometimes release stored emotional memories or sensations, given the body's role as a repository for emotional experiences. Recognizing your feelings can prepare you to handle whatever comes up during the exercises, providing a safe mental space to explore these emotions.

Practical Considerations

5. Hydration and Comfort

Ensure you are well-hydrated before beginning your exercises, as good hydration supports optimal muscle function and overall health. Also, wear comfortable clothing that allows unrestricted movement and a full range of motion during exercises.

By adopting mindful practices, setting intentions, ensuring physical readiness through gentle movements and breath control, and acknowledging your emotional state, you create an optimal environment for the body and mind to engage in the deep, healing work that Somatic exercises offer.

Basic Pandiculation Technique

Pandiculation is a core technique in Somatic exercises, a method I advocate for its profound impact on the body's sensory-motor systems. This technique is particularly significant in the context of trauma recovery and stress management. Here, I will guide you through the three essential stages of pandiculation: voluntary muscle contraction, slow and controlled muscle release, and complete relaxation.

Stage One: Voluntary Muscle Contraction

The first stage of pandiculation involves a conscious and deliberate contraction of the muscle or muscle group targeted in the exercise. This contraction is not about exerting maximum force but rather about engaging the muscles gently and mindfully to a comfortable level of tension. The purpose of this action is multifaceted:

- **Enhancing Awareness:** By voluntarily contracting the muscle, you heighten your body's awareness of that specific muscle group, which is crucial for re-establishing a connection between the brain and muscles that may have been disrupted by chronic tension or trauma.

- **Priming the Nervous System:** This controlled tension sends a clear signal to your central nervous system, indicating the current state of the muscle in terms of length and tension. This feedback is vital for the recalibration that follows.

In practice, start by gently tightening the muscle, focusing on the sensation and changes you observe. Hold the contraction for a few seconds, ensuring that you remain comfortable and mindful of your body's responses without crossing into strain.

Stage Two: Slow and Controlled Muscle Release

Following the contraction, the second stage transitions into a slow and controlled release of the muscle. This stage is crucial and should be executed with great care and attention:

- **Gradual Release:** Slowly ease the muscle out of the contraction. This gradual process allows the brain to track the change in muscle length and tension continuously, updating its sensory map of the muscle's state.

- **Neuromuscular Feedback:** As you release the muscle, maintain your focus on the sensations that accompany the lengthening. This awareness is key to retraining your brain to recognize and maintain healthier muscle tension levels without the reflexive tightening that often accompanies quick or unconscious movements.

The control with which you release the muscle tension plays a critical role in the effectiveness of pandiculation. It's not only about relaxation but about actively engaging the brain in a learning process about the muscle's new state of being.

Stage Three: Complete Relaxation

The final stage of pandiculation is complete relaxation. After the muscle has been actively contracted and carefully released, allow it to fully rest:

- **Deep Relaxation:** Encourage the muscle to relax completely, feeling the contrast between the initial tension and its new, relaxed state. This relaxation should feel deeper than the typical rest state of the muscle, given the heightened neuromuscular activity that preceded it.

- **Integration:** This stage allows the central nervous system to integrate the new information about the muscle's capacity for relaxation. It's a crucial phase for resetting the muscle's baseline tension level.

During this stage, breathe deeply and remain attentive to any residual sensations in the muscle. The complete relaxation phase is not only a release but also a powerful moment of integration and healing, allowing the body to recalibrate and retain this new state of muscular ease.

HEAD, NECK, AND SHOULDERS RELEASE

The head, neck, and shoulders are common repositories for stress and anxiety, often resulting in discomfort that can limit motion and affect our overall well-being. They are interconnected structures that support not only the physical weight of the head but also bear the brunt of psychological stress.

The muscles in these areas are prone to tightening and shortening in response to mental and emotional strain, leading to a cycle of discomfort and decreased mobility. By engaging in Somatic exercises, we can consciously interact with these muscle groups, encouraging them to relax and lengthen.

The exercises featured in this section are crafted to guide you through gentle movements and mindful awareness practices that reconnect you with your body's natural rhythms and capabilities.

Each exercise is a step towards not only physical relief but also a deeper understanding of the body's response to stress and trauma. By practicing these techniques, you engage in a form of internal exploration and healing, retraining your muscles and your mind to recognize and reduce tension.

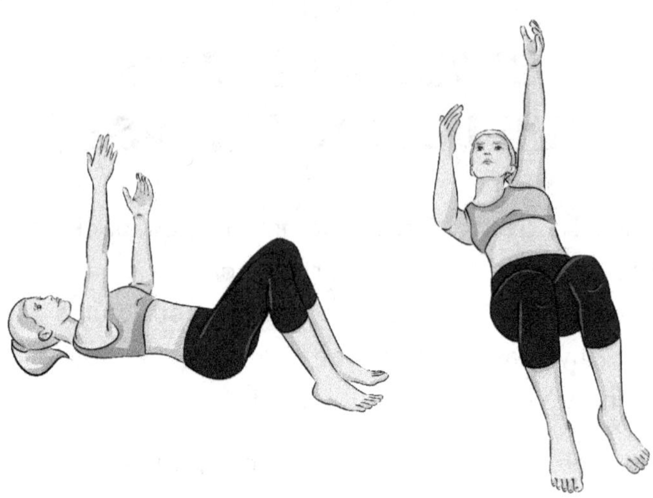

01 **Position Yourself Comfortably:** Begin by lying on your back with your knees bent and feet flat against the floor, hip-width apart. Ensure your spine is in a neutral position, and your arms are at your sides to begin.

02 **Initiate Arm Movement:** Gently raise both arms towards the ceiling, keeping them straight. Your palms should face each other, aligned with your shoulders.

03 **Engage in Alternating Reaches:** Begin with your right arm, reaching upwards as if grasping for a rope. Stretch as far as is comfortably possible, allowing your shoulder blade to move away from your spine smoothly. Slowly return to the starting position and repeat the motion 3-4 times, focusing on the stretch and movement of your shoulder.

04 **Switch to the Left Arm:** After completing the right side, switch to your left arm. Perform the same reaching motion, noticing the

subtle variations in movement and flexibility compared to your right arm. Let your right shoulder naturally counterbalance the motion by pulling back slightly as you reach with your left.

05 **Alternate Between Arms:** Continue by alternating reaches between your right and left arms. Engage each arm slowly and deliberately, noticing the interconnected movement between your shoulders and ribs. Allow your head and neck to move naturally with the motion, following the direction of your gaze upwards and back. Do this for 10 reps, 5 on each side.

06 **Add Hip Engagement:** Enhance the stretch by incorporating your hips. As you reach up with your right arm, simultaneously press down through your right foot and lift your right hip. Return to neutral and repeat on the left side. This action creates a smooth, rolling motion that helps open the ribs further and enhances the overall stretch. You can repeat this for 5 reps per side.

This exercise offers several physical benefits that contribute to both muscular and postural health:

- **Enhanced Shoulder Flexibility and Mobility:** Regularly performing this stretch increases the range of motion and flexibility in the shoulders and upper back.

- **Reduction in Upper Body Tension:** This exercise helps to release tension in the shoulders, neck, and upper back, areas often affected by stress and poor posture.

- **Increased Proprioceptive Awareness:** Engaging in controlled, mindful movements enhances body awareness, helping you to maintain better alignment and posture throughout daily activities.

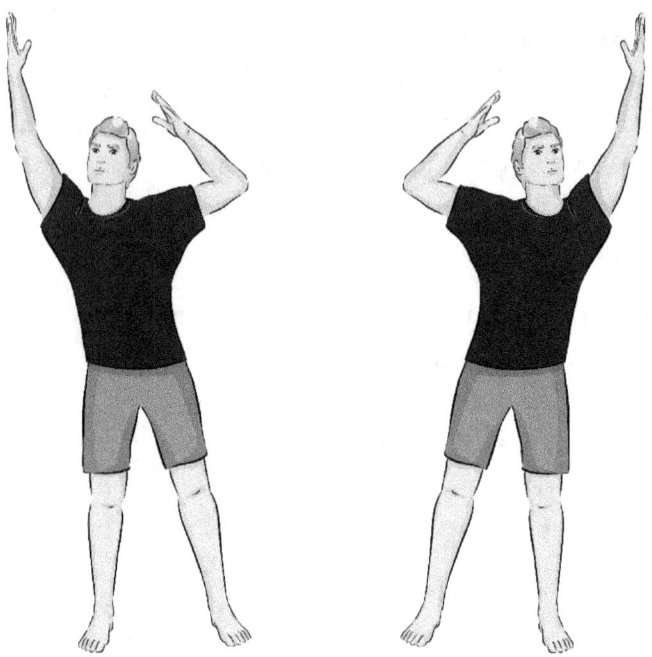

01 **Start in a Standing Position:** Stand comfortably with your feet hip-width apart. Ensure your spine is neutral, and your shoulders are relaxed, allowing your arms to hang naturally at your sides.

02 **Engage in the Initial Reach:** Imagine there is an item you need on a high shelf. Instead of only using your arm, engage your whole body. Begin by reaching upward with your right arm. As you reach, allow the left side of your body to naturally contract, pulling your left hip slightly upward.

03 **Roll onto the Ball of Your Foot:** As you reach with your right arm, roll onto the ball of your left foot. This motion helps elongate the right side of your body more effectively, enhancing the stretch from your hip to your fingertips.

04   **Return to Starting Position:** Gently return to your initial standing position, allowing your arm to come down slowly and your foot to flatten back on the ground. Take a moment to feel the release of tension in your stretched muscles.

05   **Repeat on the Opposite Side:** Now, perform the same reaching movement with your left arm, contracting the right side of your body and rolling onto the ball of your right foot. Focus on creating a balanced stretch similar to the first side.

06   **Alternate and Continue:** Continue to alternate reaches, gradually increasing the range of motion as your body becomes more comfortable with the stretch. Ensure each movement is slow and controlled, synchronizing your breathing with your reaches. You can repeat up to 10 times, 5 on each side. This is a safe exercise that you can do as long as it is comfortable.

Benefits of the Top Shelf Reach

The Top Shelf Reach not only targets the arms and shoulders but also engages the waist muscles, hips, and even the legs, offering a full-body stretch and strength experience. It is particularly beneficial for:

- **Activating and Balancing Waist Muscles:** Regular practice helps balance muscle tension on both sides of the body, which can be crucial for those who perform repetitive one-sided activities or have experienced one-sided injuries.

- **Increasing Flexibility and Ease in Daily Movements:** The comprehensive stretch provided by this exercise makes daily activities such as reaching, bending, and twisting easier and more comfortable.

- **Encouraging Healthy Posture:** Engaging the entire body in a balanced way promotes a more aligned and healthy posture, reducing the risk of imbalance-related discomfort or injury.

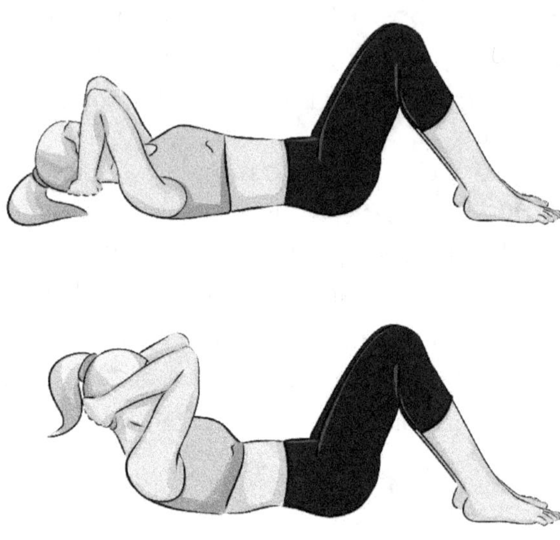

01 **Position Your Body Correctly:** Start by lying flat on your back on a comfortable surface, such as a yoga mat. Ensure your knees are bent and your feet are planted firmly on the ground, hip-width apart. Place your hands gently behind your head to support your neck.

02 **Initiate the Pull:** With your elbows pointing straight, gently pull your head upwards using your hands as support. As you lift, feel a gentle stretch along the cervical vertebrae without straining. Hold for 3 seconds.

03 **Engage in a Controlled Release:** Slowly lower your head back down to the starting position. Let your head gradually rest on the

floor ensuring the movement is smooth and controlled. Melt into the floor as you descend.

04 **Repeat the Movement:** Perform this pull and release motion 6 times, focusing on slow, mindful movements. Ensure that each lift and release cycle is performed with intentional control to maximize the stretch and relaxation of the neck muscles.

Benefits of the Head Pull and Release

This exercise is particularly beneficial for those suffering from tension headaches, neck stiffness, or the effects of prolonged forward head posture, which is increasingly common in today's digital age. Here are some specific benefits:

- **Relieves Neck Tension:** Regular practice helps alleviate the chronic tightness in the neck muscles, which often contributes to headaches and migratory pain across the shoulder blades.

- **Improves Neck Mobility:** By gently stretching and releasing the neck muscles, this exercise increases the range of motion and flexibility, which can help counteract the stiffness associated with long hours of sitting or screen time.

- **Reduces Cervical Discomfort:** The controlled lifting and lowering motion aids in decompressing the cervical vertebrae, potentially easing discomfort associated with disc issues or nerve compression.

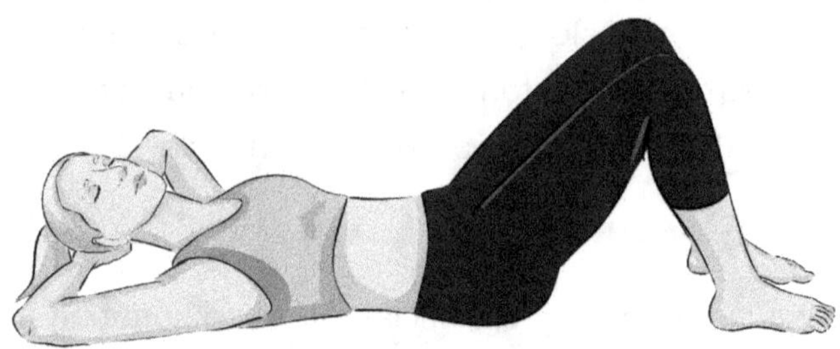

01 **Begin in a Relaxed Lying Position**: Lie down on your back on a yoga mat or a comfortable surface. Ensure your knees are bent with feet flat on the ground, hip-width apart. Place your hands behind your head to provide support without exerting pressure.

02 **Side Tilt:** Slowly tilt your head to the right side, bringing your ear closer to your shoulder. Keep the movement gentle and within a comfortable range, ensuring not to lift your shoulder towards your ear.

03 **Controlled Return:** Gradually bring your head back to the center, focusing on the natural alignment of your neck with your spine. The movement should be smooth, allowing the muscles on the side of your neck to stretch and relax naturally.

04 **Switch Sides:** Repeat the tilt on the left side, slowly bringing your left ear towards your shoulder. Ensure equal and symmetrical movement to maintain balance in muscle engagement and flexibility.

05 **Continuous Flow:** Continue this side-to-side motion for 8 repetitions. With each tilt, pause briefly to enhance the stretch on each side of your neck before returning to the center.

06 **Full Relaxation:** After completing the movements, allow your head to rest back in the neutral position on the ground. Breathe deeply and relax any remaining tension in your neck and shoulders.

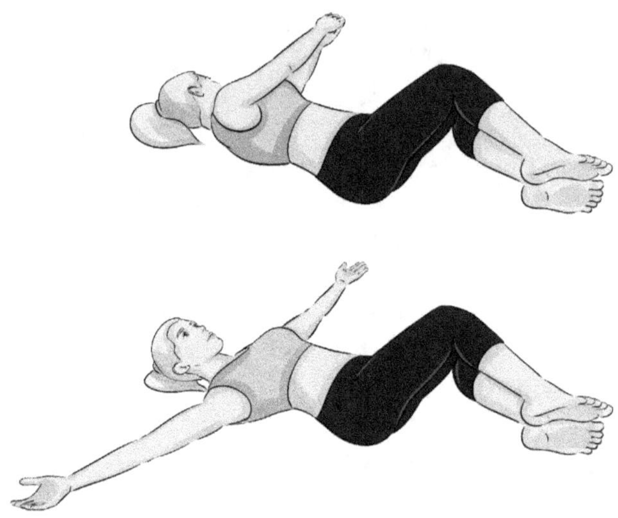

01   **Start in a Lying Position:** Begin by lying on your left side on a comfortable mat. Ensure your knees are bent with your hands clasped together on one side as shown in the image.

02   **Open Clock:** Move your right hand and let it guide you like a clock up and then extended onto the floor on the opposite side. Keep your left hand anchored on the floor. Imagine you are drawing a big circle. As your hand touches the floor, allow your body to relax and let go of any initial tension, particularly in the areas of your neck, shoulders, and arms.

03   **Close Clock:** Slowly circle the other way, moving your hand back to touch the other hand as you draw a big circle in the air. Repeat the previous 2 steps 3 times.

04 **Other Side:** You can change your position, now lying on your right side, and moving your left hand into a circle in the air, and then down into the ground, and back again clasping hands together. Repeat 3 times.

05 **Relax and Observe:** After completing several repetitions, allow your body to relax. Breathe deeply and observe any sensations of release, warmth, or ease in the areas you just worked.

Benefits of the Neck, Shoulders, and Hips Release

This exercise is designed to address common discomforts associated with prolonged periods of sitting or standing, particularly for those who work at desks or engage in repetitive tasks that impact posture. The benefits include:

- **Reduced Tension in Upper Body Areas:** Regular practice helps alleviate built-up tension in the neck, shoulders, and arms, regions prone to stress accumulation.

- **Improved Flexibility and Range of Motion:** By gently stretching and engaging these areas, the exercise enhances flexibility and overall range of motion.

- **Support for Better Posture:** As the muscles around the neck, shoulders, and arms become more relaxed and less tight, maintaining a good posture becomes easier and more natural.

6. Diagonal Arch and Curl

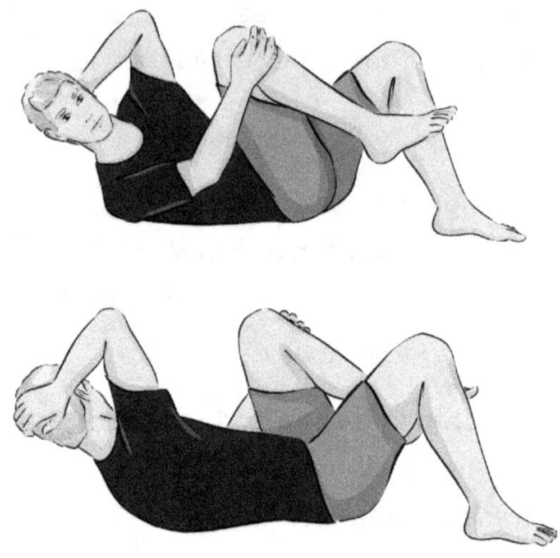

01 **Start in a Lying Position:** Begin by lying on your back on a comfortable mat. Bend your knees with feet flat on the ground.

02 **Position Your Hands and Legs:** Place your left hand behind your head and grasp your right knee with your right hand to stabilize your leg.

03 **Initiate the Arch:** Inhale deeply and gently arch your back slightly off the mat, allowing your spine to curve naturally. This helps to prepare your muscles for the curling motion.

04 **Engage in the Diagonal Curl:** As you exhale, perform a diagonal curl by bringing your left elbow towards your right knee. This movement should be controlled and focused, engaging the core muscles and obliques. Hold here for 2 seconds.

05   **Slow Return:** Slowly return to the starting position while inhaling and flattening your back against the mat. Pause momentarily to relax before the next repetition.

06   **Repeat on the Opposite Side:** Switch the positions of your hands and legs: place your right hand behind your head and hold your left knee with your left hand. Repeat the arch and diagonal curl towards the opposite side.

07   **Continue the Exercise:** Alternate sides for 8 repetitions. Focus on the smooth transition between the arch and the curl, ensuring each movement is deliberate and controlled.

Benefits of the Diagonal Arch and Curl

This exercise is designed to target multiple areas of the body, particularly the core and oblique muscles, providing several health and fitness benefits:

- **Core Strengthening**: This exercise significantly strengthens the core muscles, which improves overall stability and balance. A strong core is essential for performing a variety of daily activities and other exercises effectively.

- **Enhanced Oblique Activation**: The diagonal movement engages the oblique muscles, which are crucial for side bending and waist twisting movements. This can lead to improved waist definition and mobility.

- **Increased Spinal Flexibility**: The arching and curling motions increase the flexibility of the spine, promoting better posture and reducing the risk of back injuries.

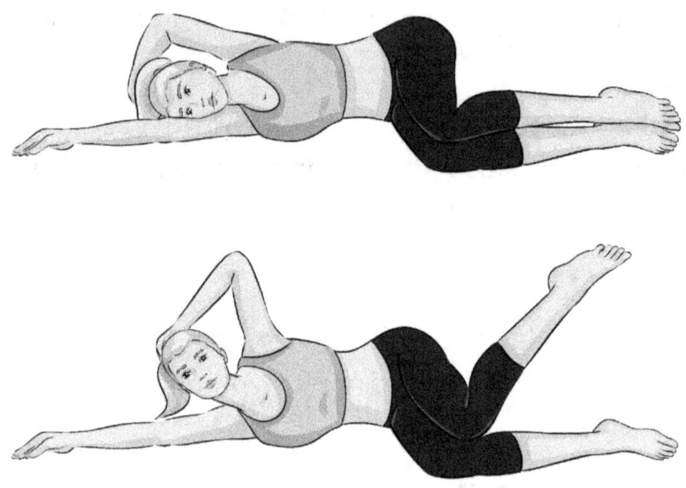

01   **Start in a Side-Lying Position:** Begin by lying on your side on a comfortable mat. Rest on your bottom arm or use an actual pillow for support. Bend your knees so they are aligned with your hips, and ensure your ankles are directly under your knees for stability.

02   **Position Your Top Arm:** Wrap your top arm over your head, gently cradling it. This arm placement helps maintain balance and aligns your body correctly for the exercise.

03   **Engage Your Obliques:** As you inhale, simultaneously lift your head with your hands and the foot of your top leg while keeping your knees together. This movement should create a contraction in your oblique muscles, bringing your hip and armpit closer together. Hold for 2 seconds.

04   **Controlled Release:** Then, slowly exhale and release your head and foot back to the starting position. Ensure the movement is controlled and gradual to maximize the pandiculation. Repeat 5 times.

05   **Switch Sides:** Switch sides and repeat the lifting and lowering movement 3 times.

06   **Rest:** Once you have completed the exercise on both sides, roll onto your back and rest for a few moments, allowing your muscles to relax and your breathing return to normal. Melt into the floor and feel your muscles completely relax.

Benefits of the Lateral Flexion Exercise

This lateral flexion exercise is particularly beneficial for several aspects of physical health and wellness:

- **Strengthens Oblique Muscles**: It targets the oblique muscles on the sides of the abdomen, essential for core stability and waist mobility.

- **Improves Flexibility**: The movement enhances the flexibility of the spine and rib cage, contributing to better overall spinal health.

- **Improves Proprioception**: Engaging in precise, controlled movements enhances your body's proprioceptive awareness, which is crucial for balance and coordinated movements.

BACK RELEASE

Our back contains muscles, nerves, and connective tissues that often bear the brunt of our daily stresses and strains. It is not just a critical component of our physical frame; it is also a repository for emotional tensions and unprocessed traumas. The exercises I present here are designed not only to relieve pain or improve flexibility but also to foster a deeper dialogue between the mind and the body.

As we explore these seven exercises for back release, each movement is crafted to gently encourage the muscles to unwind and let go of the habitual patterns that lead to stiffness and discomfort. This process is similar to unlocking a door that has been stuck for years, slowly and carefully easing out of old ways of moving and responding to our environment. Through careful attention to the nuances of bodily sensations, these exercises allow us to reconnect with parts of ourselves that may have been ignored or suppressed.

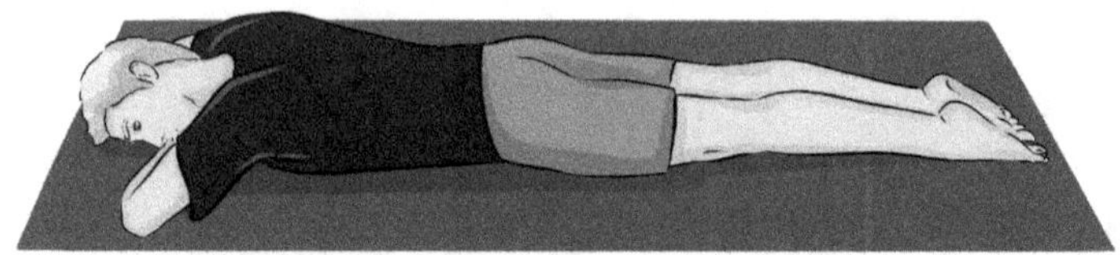

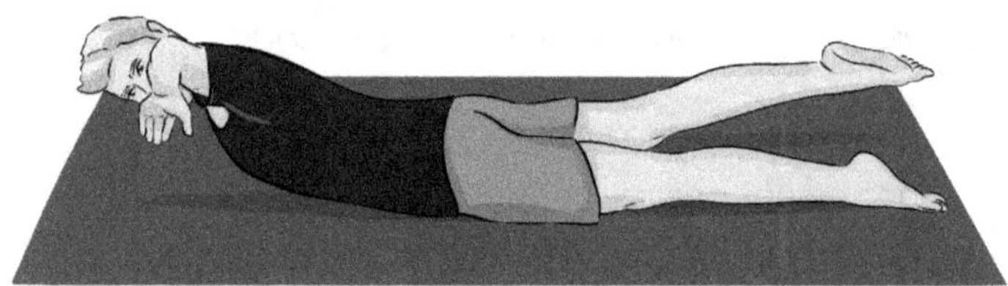

01 **Start in a Prone Position:** Begin by lying face down on a comfortable mat. Position yourself so that your body is straight and relaxed.

02 **Hand and Cheek Placement:** Place the back of your left hand under your right cheek, turning your face to the left. This alignment helps support the neck and stabilizes the spine during the extension.

03 **Initiate the Extension:** Inhale deeply and simultaneously lift your head, the elbow of the arm under your cheek, and the opposite (right) leg. Ensure that the movement is smooth and controlled, engaging the muscles along your back. Hold for 1-2 seconds depending on your flexibility and strength.

04   **Controlled Descent:** Exhale slowly as you lower your head, elbow, and leg back to the mat. Focus on the sensation of pandiculation in each muscle group relaxing as you return to the starting position. Repeat up to 5 times.

05   **Switch Sides:** After completing, switch sides by placing the back of your right hand under your left cheek. As you move up, raise your left leg. Repeat the same reps on this side to ensure balanced muscle engagement.

06   **Relaxation:** Once you have completed the exercise on both sides, relax with your tummy and melt into the floor. Allow your muscles to relax completely and your breathing to return to normal.

Benefits of the Back Extension Exercise

The back extension exercise offers numerous benefits, particularly for strengthening and mobilizing the back:

- **Strengthens Lower Back Muscles**: This exercise targets the lower back muscles, essential for supporting the spine and improving posture.

- **Enhances Spinal Health**: Regular practice of back extensions can increase spinal flexibility and reduce the risk of back injuries.

- **Improves Posture**: Strengthening the muscles along the spine helps in maintaining a proper posture, which can alleviate common issues such as back pain and muscle fatigue.

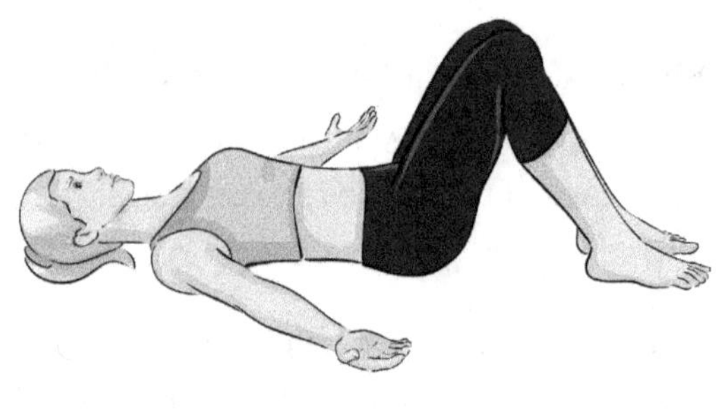

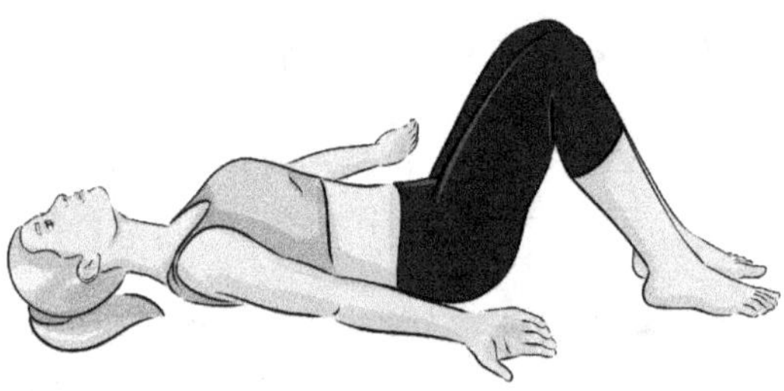

01 **Start in a Supine Position:** Begin by lying on your back with your knees bent and your feet flat on the floor. This starting position helps in maintaining the natural curve of your spine. Place your hands on your sides, palm open and up.

02 **Inhale and Arch Your Back:** As you inhale, gently arch your back, and roll your hands inward toward your stomach. You're going to feel like a twisted towel.

03 **Exhale and Flatten Your Back:** Slowly exhale and reverse the arch by flattening your back against the floor, and rolling your hands clockwise back on the floor with palms facing up. Repeat up to 6 times

04   **Awareness:** Once you finish, relax and let go of your back on the floor. Feel your body melt. Observe any lingering emotions here for up to 10 seconds as you breathe and completely relax.

Benefits of the Arch & Flatten Exercise

This exercise targets the upper body component, specifically the spinal and neck regions. The nuanced movement here promotes proprioception, the awareness of the body's position and movements. It's a bit challenging, but after the relaxation and pandiculation movements, it completely calms your nervous system, reducing stress. This is one of my favorites!

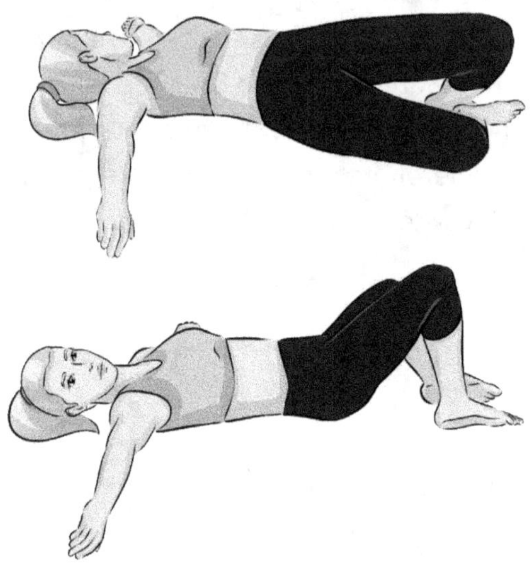

01 **Start in a Lying Position:** Lie on your back with your knees bent and feet flat on the floor. Ensure your spine is neutral and your shoulders are relaxed on the ground.

02 **Extend Your Arms:** Extend your arms out from your shoulders, forming a T-shape with your body. This position helps stabilize your upper body and allows for a full range of motion during the twist.

03 **Begin the Twist:** As you exhale, gently lower your knees to one side, keeping them together and ensuring your shoulders remain in contact with the floor. Turn your head to face the opposite direction of your knees to enhance the twist. As you move to one side, your hands will naturally rotate with the twist. Let them do so.

04   **Hold and Breathe:** Hold the twisted position for a moment, breathing deeply. Then, let go and completely turn to the other side. Notice the pandiculation in your torso, spine and arms. Go back and forth, left to right for up to 8 reps.

05   **Return to Center:** Inhale as you bring your knees and head back to the center, aligning them with your spine again. Rest here for up to a minute, relax completely, and melt into the floor.

Benefits of The Twist

The Twist is a gentle yet effective exercise designed to pandiculate your spine, arms, head and torso. It's a very effective move and can help reduce back pain.

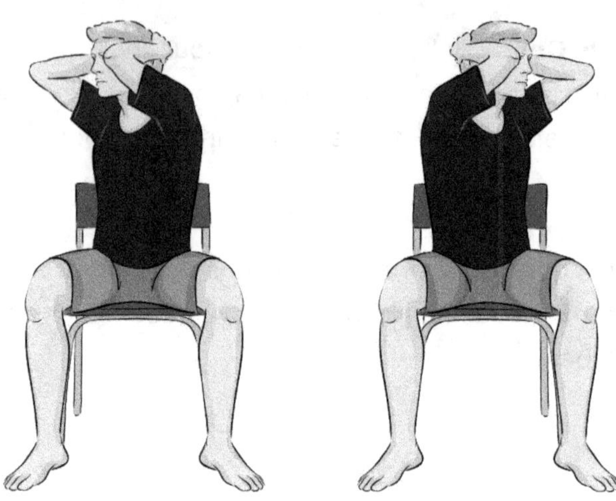

01 **Starting Position:** Sit comfortably with a straight spine and relaxed shoulders. Place your hands behind your head, interlacing your fingers for support.

02 **Align Elbows and Nose:** Ensure that your elbows are pointing forward, aligning with the direction of your nose. This alignment is crucial for maintaining the integrity of the movement throughout the exercise. Now turn back the other direction. Repeat up to 8 times. Feel the pandiculation in your back.

03 **Rotational Movement:** An optional variation is to bend downward as you turn, facing your nose, eyes and elbows 45 degrees looking at the ground behind you. This extends the pandiculation to your upper back and shoulders.

04 **Return to Center:** Slowly bring your head and elbows back to the center and rest for up to 30 seconds.

This dynamic exercise, dubbed "Rotational Realignments," is great for office workers or anytime you're stuck waiting. You can even do it without a chair. It's a lovely movement whenever you're waiting around. Sometimes, I do this while waiting in line. People ask me what I'm doing and it becomes a great conversation starter.

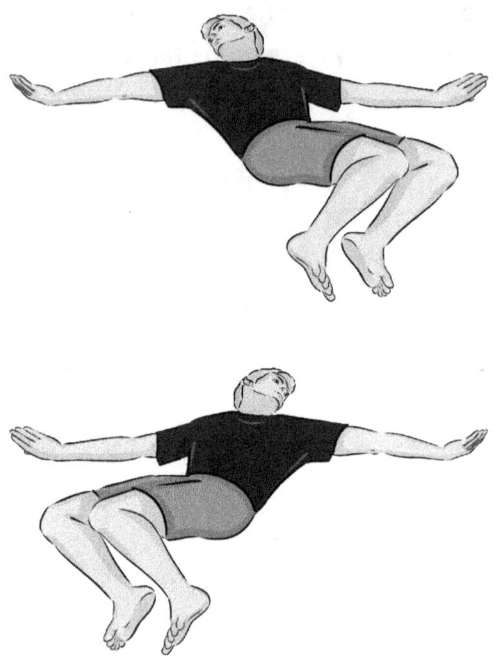

01   **Starting Position:** Lie on your back with your knees bent and feet flat on the floor, hip-width apart. Ensure your spine is in a neutral position.

02   **Washrag:** Think of yourself as a wet washrag, being wrung dry. Lower your knees to the left and at the same time turn your head to the right.

03   **Arm Positioning:** Extend your arms to the sides and open your palms naturally turning them as you move. Your hands will follow naturally as you do this. Think of wringing your body like a wet washrag.

04   **Wring:** Now turn to the other side. Lift your legs and lower them to the other side. As you do, turn your head to the other side. Keep

your arms out and turn your wrist and hands naturally as you do. Feeling clean yet? This is a beautiful movement that pandiculates your entire body when done right.

05 **Coordinate Breathing:** Inhale and exhale slowly as you move from side to side. Repeat as many times as comfortable. I do 10 rotations side to side in the morning and it feels amazing.

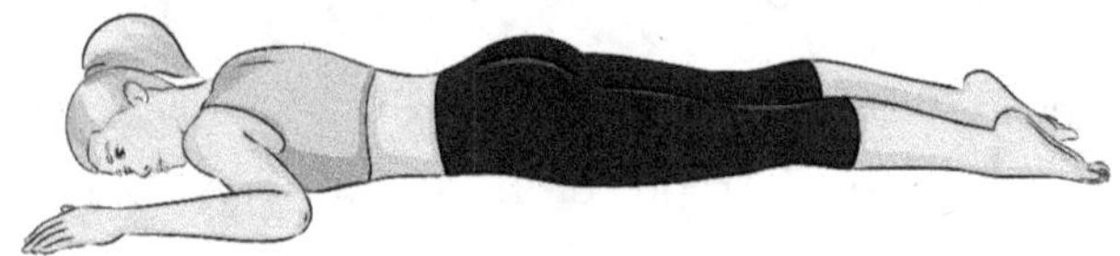

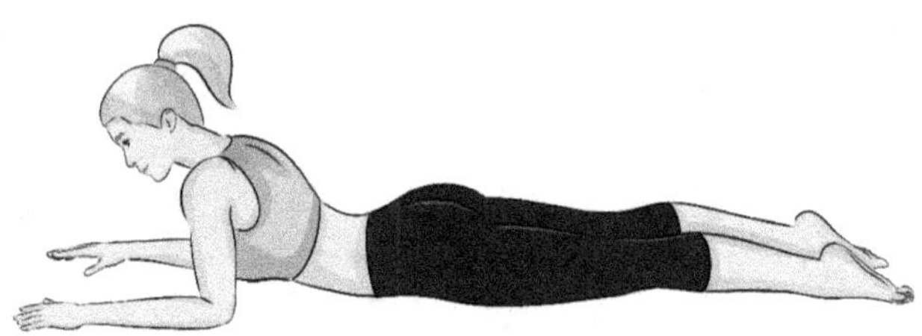

01 **Prepare Your Space:** Start by lying on your stomach on a comfortable, flat surface. Place your hands gently beside your head.

02 **Lift and Contract:** Gently lift your head to engage the muscles in your back. This is not about lifting high but rather feeling the contraction from your upper to your lower back. Keep your hands on the floor as you lift up.

03 **Pause and Feel:** Hold at the peak of your lift. This pause allows you to feel the contraction throughout your back, from the base of your skull down to your tailbone.

04 **Controlled Release:** As you exhale, slowly begin to lower your head back to the floor. This slow release is where the pandiculation magic happens, as it lets your back muscles to let go and lengthen. Repeat up to 8 times.

05 **Variation:** You can slowly turn your head to one side, increasing the muscle contraction on the opposite lower back to treat specific areas that feel tense.

The abdomen and pelvis, areas rich with visceral and muscular connections, often harbor unresolved stress and emotional turmoil, manifesting through physical stiffness and chronic discomfort. The sacral chakra and the solar plexus chakra are two chakras located in the stomach and pelvic area of the body.

Sacral chakra

Located in the lower abdomen, between the navel and the perineum, this chakra is associated with sexuality, emotions, and creativity. It's often referred to as the sexual chakra since it's connected to the reproductive organs. Some say that when this chakra is out of balance, it can lead to issues like menstrual problems, impotence, and jealousy.

Solar plexus chakra

Located in the solar plexus, between the upper abdomen and the chest bone, this chakra is associated with self-esteem, determination, and courage. It's connected to the liver, gallbladder, stomach, spleen, and pancreas. Some say that when this chakra is out of balance, it can lead to issues like digestive disorders, depression, and low energy.

The exercises I have curated for you are designed to foster an intimate dialogue between your energy, emotions and body. By consciously contracting and gently releasing these core muscles, you will learn to listen to your body. Through this intentional practice, you can expect to gain greater control over your stress responses, improve your bodily alignment and digestion, and enhance your overall sense of well-being.

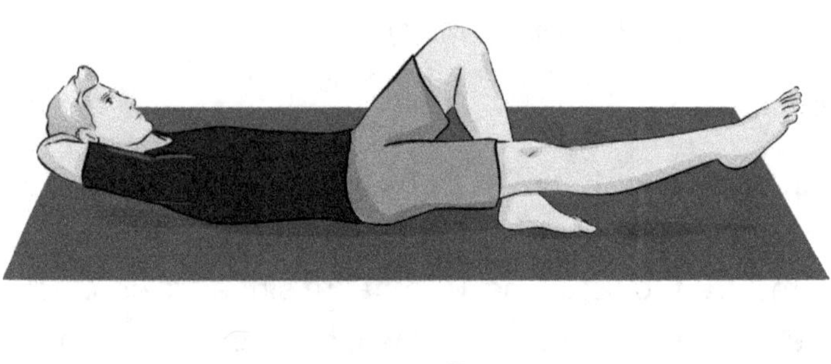

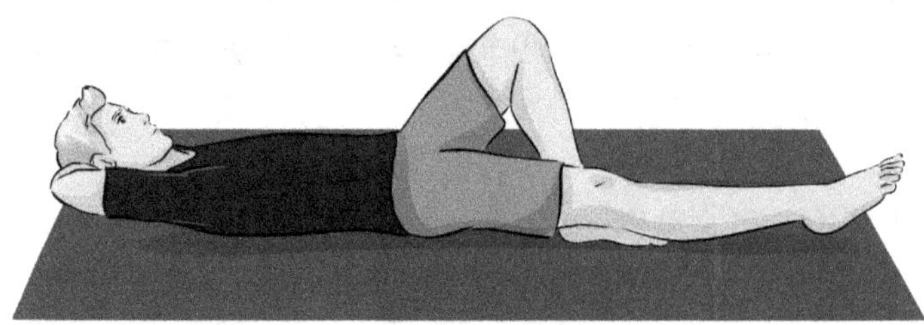

01   Find a comfortable, flat surface where you can lie down. Place a mat or a soft towel under you if necessary.

02   **Position your legs:** Bend your knees with your feet flat on the floor, spaced comfortably apart and aligned directly under your knees.

03   **Place your hands:** Bring your arms to your sides with palms facing down. Or, you can place your hands behind your head for support.

04   **Engage your psoas:** As you exhale slowly, gently extend one leg straight along the floor with your toes pointing straight, hovering just above the ground. Keep the movement slow and controlled, focusing on the sensation in your lower back and the front of your hip. Hold for 3 to 5 seconds if you can. Keep your lower back

pressed gently against the floor to ensure the psoas muscle is properly engaged during the leg extension.

05 **Return to starting position:** Slowly bring the extended leg back to the starting position as you inhale. Repeat the movement with the other leg.

06 Alternate legs for up to 8 repetitions, focusing on the smoothness and control of the movement. Breathe deeply and consistently throughout the exercise. Stop at any time if you feel discomfort or pain. If you cannot hold for more than 3 seconds, lower it to 1 second and start slow.

Benefits of the Psoas Release

- The psoas muscles are often unseen culprits in pelvic pain, lower body instability and loss of balance. This exercise helps you release them without strenuous trigger point work or exercise

- This particular movement works wonders when combined with a deep tissue masseuse who can help you release tense muscles along the lower back, abdominal area and pelvic area. During my healing from pelvic pain, this was one of the core exercises to help me regain my strength.

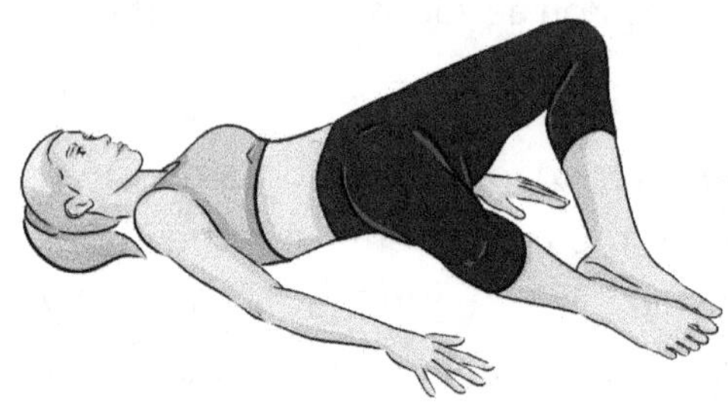

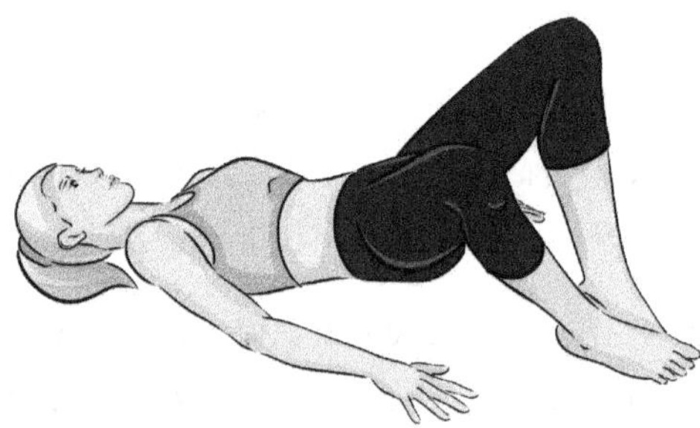

01 **Begin in a relaxed position:** Lie down on your back on a flat, comfortable surface such as a yoga mat. Ensure you have enough space around you to extend your arms and legs freely.

02 **Position your legs:** Bend your knees with your feet flat on the ground, positioned hip-width apart. This stabilizes your lower body and prepares you for the exercise.

03 **Arm placement:** Extend your arms outward to the sides, palms facing down. This alignment helps maintain balance

04 **Initiate the pelvic tilt:** Engage your core and pelvic floor muscles by slightly lifting your pelvis off the floor. Hold this lifted position for a few seconds to activate the core muscles fully. Think of yourself pulling your pelvic floor upwards.

05   **Let go:** Lower your pelvis back to the floor gradually. Ensure your movements are slow and controlled to maximize the pandiculation of your abdominal and pelvic muscles. Repeat for up to 5 times.

Benefits of the Pelvic Floor Release:

- **Improves Core Stability:** Regularly performing this exercise enhances the strength and stability of your core muscles, which support proper posture and spinal alignment.

- **Enhances Pelvic Floor Function:** This exercise promotes the relaxation and strengthening of the pelvic floor muscles, which is beneficial for bladder and bowel function.

- **Relieves Stress and Tension:** The focused, gentle movements help to reduce physical stress and tension, particularly in the pelvic region, which can be beneficial for overall mental well-being.

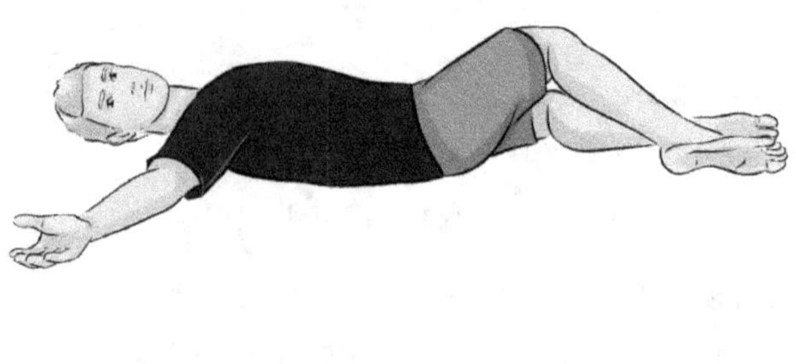

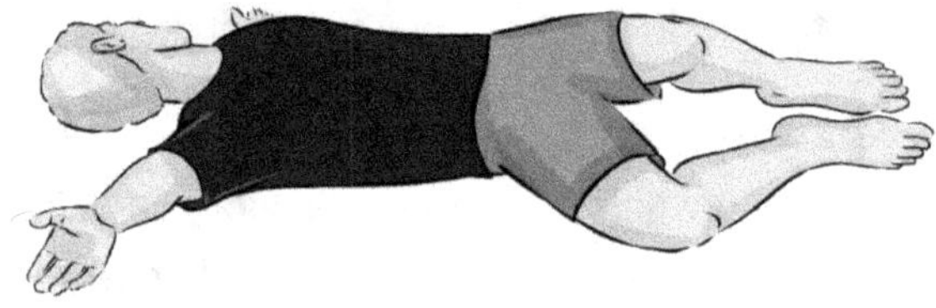

01   **Begin in a relaxed position:** Lie on your back on a comfortable surface. Put your knees together as you lift them up, with feet flat on the floor and your arms extended.

02   **Controlled turn:** Let your legs bend to one side, while your head turns to the opposite side. Let your arms turn naturally as you do this. You should feel a pandiculation of your torso and mid-body as you turn. Lovely! Isn't it?

03   **Return and repeat:** Slowly go from side to side. I usually do 10 in the morning, 5 toward each side. This is an easier version of the washrag and requires less flexibility. It also targets your mid torso with more focus.

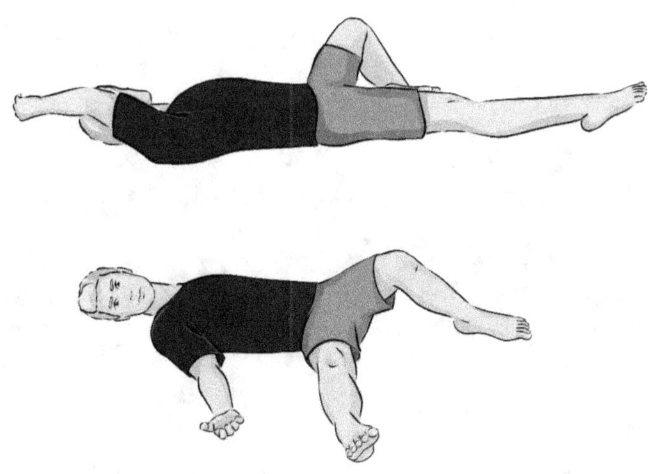

01 **Setup and initial relaxation:** Lie on your back and extend your arms out to the side and legs straight.

02 **Find your rotation:** Imagine your right arm as the dial on a clock. You're going from 12 to 9 o'clock with your right arm and your right leg as well.

03 **Rotate:** Now, rotate your right arm from 9 o'clock to 2 or 3 o'clock, as far as you can. At the same time, bring your right leg to 6 o'clock. Your left leg can bend naturally following your right arm, the clock dial. Now go back and forth up to 4 times.

04 **Reverse the dial:** Next, use your left arm as the dial, and reverse positions. Start at 12 and go down to 3 o'clock, then back to 9 or 10 o'clock. Repeat this up to 4 times.

05 **Increase range of motion:** As you do these circular movements, go slowly to trigger pandiculation. Your range of motion will increase too.

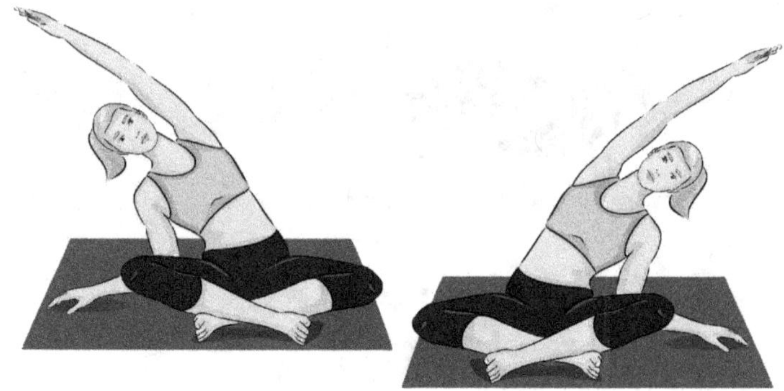

01 **Starting Position:** Sit comfortably and cross your legs. Take a few breaths. This is a good time to do a brief body scan.

02 **Engage Core and Stretch:** Begin by raising your right arm and extend to the left. Keep your left hand on the floor for stability.

03 **Fluid Motion to Opposite Side:** Return to the center, and now raise your left arm to the right. Allow your breath to guide the movement, ensuring a smooth and controlled pace.

04 **Deepen the Stretch:** Continue alternating sides for up to 10 repetitions. With each repetition, try to deepen the stretch slightly more without compromising the form. As you return, go slowly to trigger the pandiculation response.

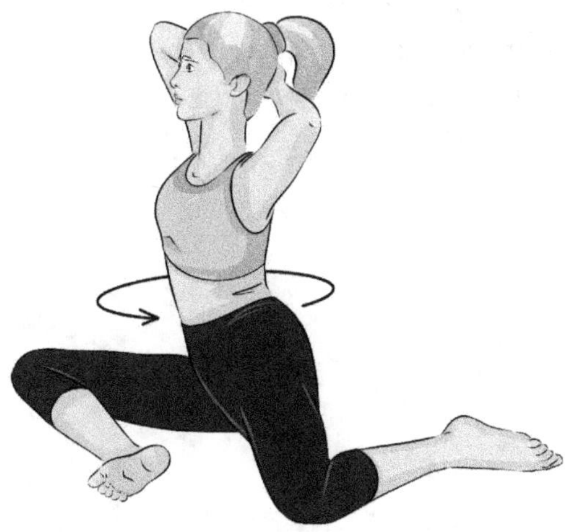

01   **Start:** Place your right leg in front of you, foot facing outward and your left leg behind you, feet pointing back as shown in the picture above.

02   **Stability:** Place both of your hands behind your head for stability as you do the hip circles. Slowly turn your hips in a clockwise direction.

03   **Deepen the Hip Circles:** Gradually increase the range of motion of your hip circles, ensuring that your movement remains smooth and rhythmic. Do 5 circles.

04   **Switch rotation:** Then, turn the other direction, counterclockwise for 5 reps.

05   **Switch position:** Now, reverse your legs position and repeat the previous steps, with your left leg forward and right leg back. Repeat the clockwise and counter-clockwise circles slowly for 10 reps total.

Tip: As you perform Hip Circles, visualize drawing a perfect circle with your hips. This mental imagery encourages a full range of motion and symmetrical movement, which helps evenly distribute the mobility work across all surrounding muscles. Ensure the movement is fluid and continuous, akin to stirring a gentle cauldron, to prevent any jerky motions that could lead to muscle strain.

LOWER BODY RELEASE

The lower body acts as the foundation of our being. Just as a house relies on its foundation to remain stable, our bodies depend on a resilient lower body to navigate movements and balance. The exercises presented here are crafted to enhance flexibility, build balance awareness, improve circulation, and reduce stiffness.

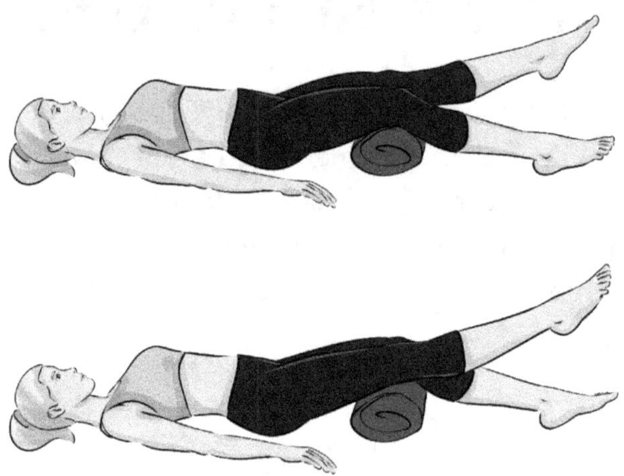

01 **Begin by preparing your space:** Lay a yoga mat on the floor and position a bolster or a stack of firm pillows at one end. If you do not have a bolster, large, tightly rolled towels or a thick blanket will suffice. The aim is to create a supportive platform that can elevate your legs comfortably.

02 **Position yourself on the mat:** Lie down on your back with your legs extended. Slide towards the bolster so that when you bend your knees, your lower legs can rest comfortably on the bolster with your knees pointing upwards. This alignment helps decompress the spine and allows the quadriceps to relax.

03 **Begin the quadriceps release:** With your legs supported by the bolster, focus on one leg at a time. Gradually attempt to straighten

the knee, pushing your heel towards the ceiling. It's crucial to move within a range that feels comfortable and pain-free.

04 **Hold the extension briefly:** Once you have extended your leg as much as comfortably possible, hold the position to intensify the stretch across the thigh. Ensure that you maintain a smooth breathing pattern to help deepen the relaxation.

05 **Slowly release the stretch:** Gently lower the leg back onto the bolster, allowing the muscles to relax progressively. The slow movement encourages the nervous system to release tension deeply embedded within the muscle fibers.

06 **Rotate the leg for medial and lateral focus:** To specifically target the medial and lateral quadriceps, slightly rotate your leg inward and outward as you perform the stretch. Inward rotation focuses more on the lateral (outer) quadriceps, while outward rotation targets the medial (inner) quadriceps.

07 **Repeat on the other leg:** After completing the sequence on one leg, switch to the other leg and repeat the entire process to ensure balanced muscle relaxation.

08 **Conclude with relaxation:** After stretching both legs, rest with your legs on the bolster for a few minutes. Use this time to breathe deeply and allow your entire body to relax, facilitating a deep integration of the exercise's benefits.

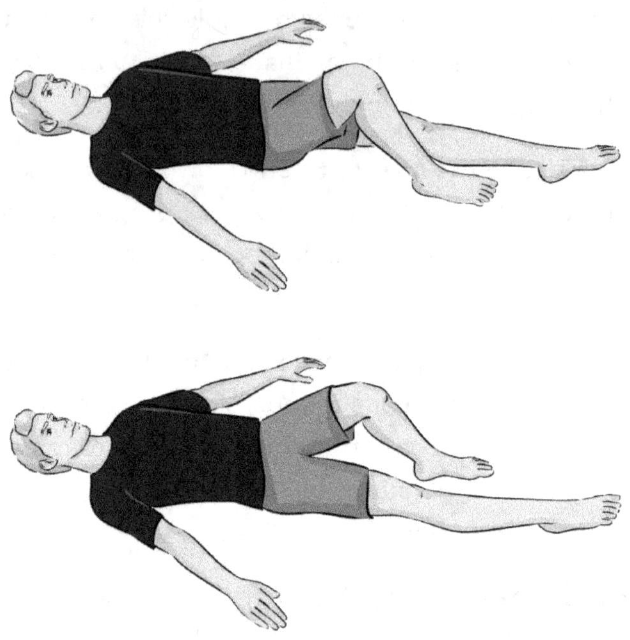

01   Lay down a yoga mat or place a towel on the floor. Put both hands extended 45-degrees on the floor, palms down

02   Shift one knee up and tighten your hamstrings as you do. You should feel a tightening on the back of your hamstring/leg area.

03   Take a breath and then slowly release, triggering the pandiculation of your back leg/hamstring area. Repeat up to 6 times.

04   Repeat with the other leg for up to 6 reps.

05   Take a few breaths and notice your emotions. Sink your legs back into the floor, totally relaxed. Stay there for a few breaths before going onto the next movement.

22. Reverse Lower Back Release

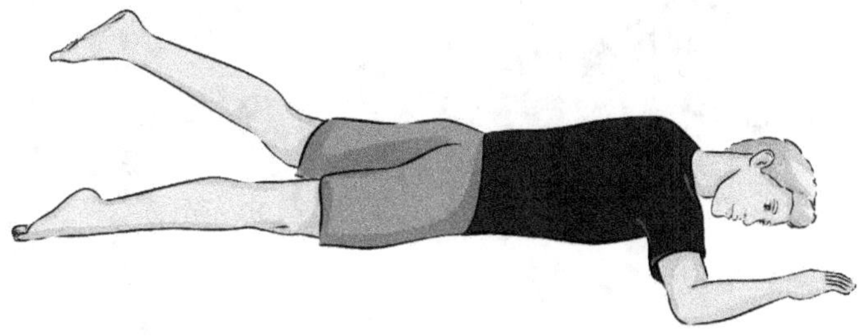

01   Begin by lying flat with your stomach on a comfortable surface, such as a yoga mat. Ensure that your body is aligned straight, with your arms resting naturally by your head, palm on the floor. Allow your forehead to gently rest on the mat or a folded towel to keep your neck aligned.

02   Slowly raise one leg and go as high as you can. If this gets difficult, just raise it to a level that feels comfortable for you now.

03   After holding for 2 seconds, slowly lower it with controlled resistance. This will trigger the pandiculation effect. You should feel muscle contraction in your lower back, buttocks, and back hamstrings.

04   Repeat for 5 reps. Then do the same with the other leg.

05   Focus on breathing deeply and relaxing during each stretch. Pay attention to your breathing, inhaling deeply as you prepare to lift your leg, and exhaling as you release. This focus on breath helps in reducing tension and promoting relaxation throughout the exercise.

06   You can hold your leg longer or release it slower to trigger a strong pandiculation response.

23. Quadriceps Release

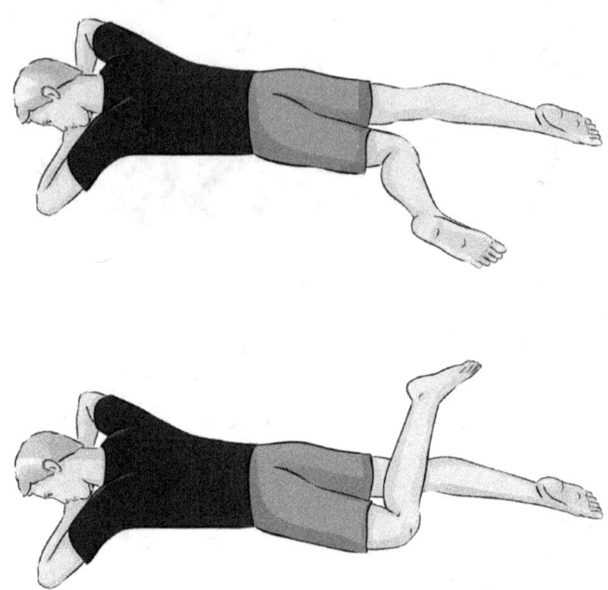

01   Start by lying flat on your stomach with your hands holding your face on a yoga mat or soft surface. You can start with your head turned left, hands resting against your right cheek.

02   Raise your left leg again and turn it slowly from 12 to 9 o'clock (outward from body). Keep the movement controlled and focused on the sensation in your thigh. You should feel pandiculation in the left oblique muscles and lower back.

03   Now raise your left leg 90 degrees, then turn it clockwise from 12 to 3 o'clock (legs moving inward). Slowly lower the leg to trigger the pandiculation effect. You should feel pandiculation in the left leg and lower back while the side of your body is tensing and relaxing. Repeat this 3 times.

04   Repeat the movement with your right leg for up to 3 times.

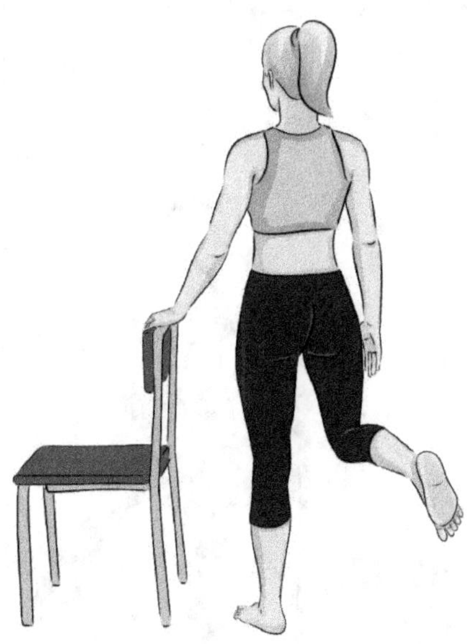

01 Start by standing comfortably next to a sturdy chair or surface for support. Your spine should be elongated, and shoulders relaxed. Use the chair to maintain balance and ensure you do not strain during the exercise.

02 Place one hand on the support and gently lift one foot off the floor at a 90-degree angle. Slowly and with control, extend the lifted leg backward. Keep your supporting leg slightly bent (not locked in straight) at the knee to maintain flexibility

03 Hold for 1 to 2 seconds and release downward. You should feel pandiculation in the lower hamstrings and calf muscles. Repeat this 5 times.

04 Switch hands for stability and raise the opposite leg. Again, repeat this for up to 5 times.

05 Throughout the exercise, keep your breathing steady and deep. Keep the muscles of your neck and shoulders relaxed to prevent any tension, as we focus on pandiculation in the legs.

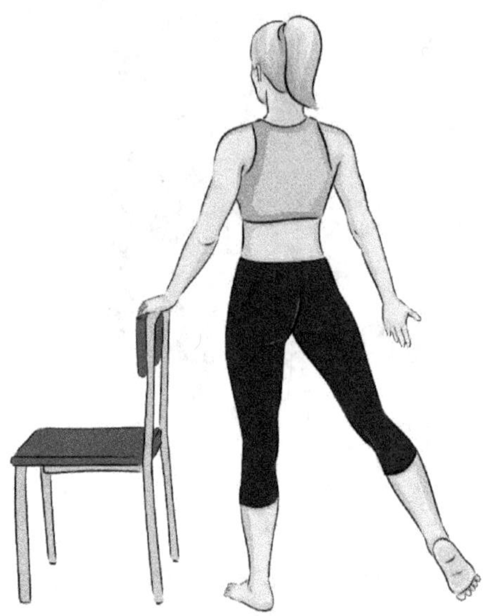

01   Begin by standing next to a stable support such as a chair or a wall. Place one hand on the support for balance. Ensure your spine is elongated and your shoulders are relaxed to maintain proper posture.

02   Slowly extend your right leg outward while keeping it straight. Hold for 3 seconds and then slowly return to standing position. You should feel a trigger in pandiculation on the lower hamstring area. Repeat this for 4 reps.

03   Now, repeat this with the left leg for 4 reps, focusing on slow, controlled movements.

FOOT EXERCISES

As a Somatic educator, a health practitioner, and a former professional athlete, I've seen firsthand how the subtleties of foot health can echo through the entire body, influencing posture, mobility, and even mental state.

Here, we delve into a series of exercises designed to enhance your awareness of these crucial yet often neglected parts of our bodies. These exercises are not merely routines; they are gateways to discovering how deeply our feet are integrated with the sensory experiences of our lives.

Each movement and stretch I've outlined here is more than a physical task; it is a step towards reprogramming the sensory pathways that have been muted by the monotonous use or restrictive footwear.

By engaging with these exercises, you will begin to peel back layers of tension and restriction, allowing for a fuller sense of relief that can ripple upward, potentially easing discomforts that may even extend to areas far from your feet.

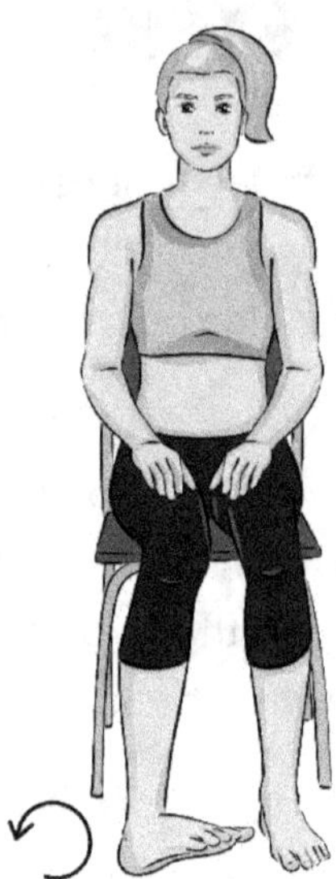

01   Begin with a comfortable seated position. Sit in a chair with your feet flat on the floor. Make sure your spine is elongated and your shoulders are relaxed. Adjust your setting as necessary to ensure comfort and proper posture.

02   Focus on one leg at a time to isolate the exercise. Start with either leg, ensuring that the other foot remains flat on the floor to maintain balance and stability.

03   Gently begin to raise your foot and turn it slowly in one direction. Hold for 2 seconds, and slowly return to center. You should feel pandiculation in the upper part of your feet.

04 Then, rotate your foot in the opposite direction (clockwise or counterclockwise), and release slowly as you return to the center. Repeat the motion as often as you like.

05 Now try with the other foot. You should feel both feet getting lighter and less tight after this movement.

27. Gentle Foot Activation from a Supine Position

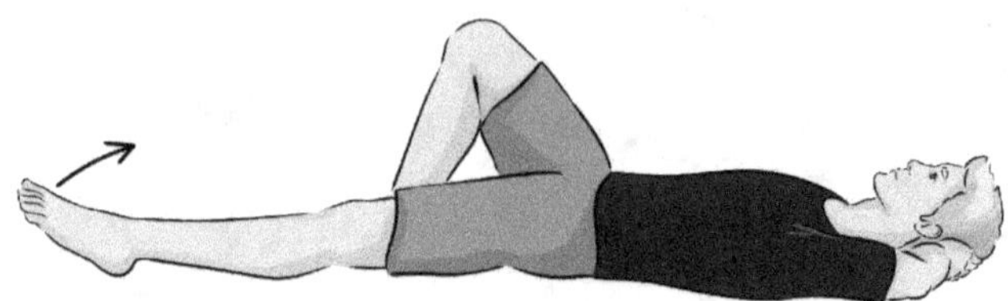

01   **Lie down on a comfortable surface with your back flat.** Relax and ensure your spine is naturally aligned, arms resting behind your head.

02   **Start with one leg extended and the other leg bent at the knee.** The bent knee will help stabilize your body during the exercise, maintaining focus on the working leg.

03   **Flex the foot of your extended leg by drawing the toes back toward your shin.** This movement engages the muscles along your shin and stretches the calf muscles.

04   **Now point the toes of your extended leg away from you.** Focus on creating a smooth, controlled movement, extending through the ball of your foot to activate the calf muscles fully.

05   **The extension triggers pandiculation in the upper foot.** The flex upon release triggers pandiculation in the front lower leg area.

06   **Repeat the flexing and pointing 3-4 times.** Ensure a rhythmic pattern, holding each position briefly to maximize muscle engagement.

07   **Switch to your other foot and perform the same sequence.** This ensures both legs work equally, maintaining balance in muscle strength and flexibility.

08 **Introduce slight variations by rotating the ankle.** Rotate inward and outward to engage different aspects of the ankle and calf muscles, enhancing overall mobility.

09 **Finish by resting briefly and then repeating the sequence.** Allow your muscles to relax completely before starting the next exercise.

Benefits of Gentle Foot Activation:

- **Increases Circulation:** This exercise helps to boost blood flow to your lower extremities, which is beneficial for overall foot health and can aid in faster recovery from foot-related ailments.

- **Enhances Foot and Ankle Flexibility:** Regular performance improves the flexibility of the foot and ankle, reducing the risk of injuries during daily activities or exercise.

- **Strengthens Foot Muscles:** Activating the muscles in the foot helps in building strength, which can improve balance, gait, and athletic performance.

- **Relieves Foot Tension:** This exercise can help alleviate tension and pain in the feet, particularly beneficial for those who stand for long periods or have conditions like plantar fasciitis.

- **Improves Neuromuscular Coordination:** Engaging the foot in various movements enhances coordination between the nerves and muscles, improving your ability to perform complex movements with greater ease.

> **Tip:** While lying on your back, keep your legs straight and relaxed on the ground. As you gently flex and point your feet, maintain a rhythm that feels natural and not forced. This exercise is about awakening the nerve endings in your feet without straining the muscles. Focus on the smooth transition between movements to increase circulation and awareness in your feet.

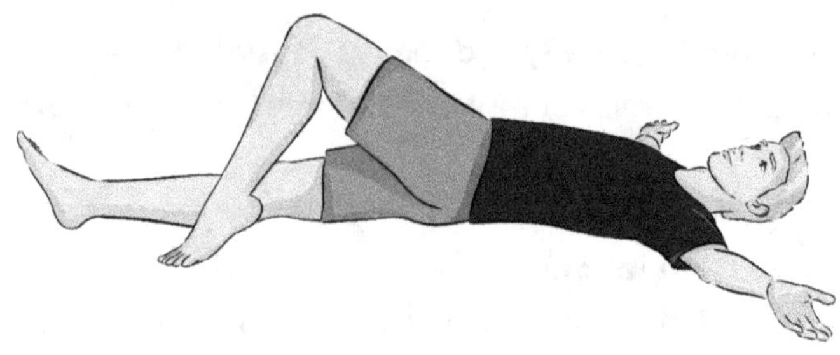

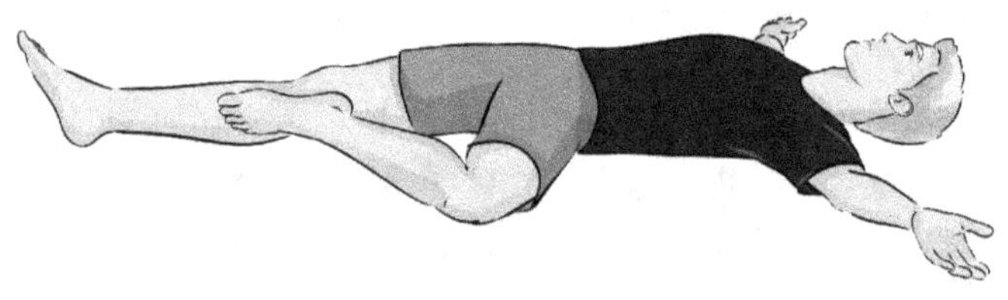

01   **Begin by lying flat on your back with your arms at your sides.** Ensure your spine is naturally aligned and relaxed on a firm, flat surface.

02   **Bend one knee and extend your toes upward as much as you can. Slowly lift your pelvis off the ground, engaging your core and glute muscles.** Keep the lift gentle, focusing on the control and alignment of your hips. **Your head will naturally turn to the opposite side of the leg (raise right leg, head turns left). Hold for a second then slowly release downward. Do up to 3 reps.**

03   Now, allow your knee and leg to gently lower to the floor. As you do, you will feel pandiculation of the inner adductor muscles (upper leg). Repeat up to 3 times.

04   **Now repeat for the other side for up to 3 reps going each side.**

05   **Complete the session with a moment of relaxation.** Lie flat with your legs extended and arms by your sides, allowing your body to fully absorb the benefits of the exercise.

Benefits of Gentle Pelvic Lifts for Foot Release:

This exercise can reduce pain and stiffness in lower leg muscles and the foot. Combined with trigger point work, this often reduces stress on daily movement and activities.

- **Increases Circulation in Lower Extremities:** The movement helps boost blood flow to the legs and feet, which can reduce swelling and improve foot health.

- **Relieves Foot Pressure:** By alternating foot pressure, the exercise can help distribute and reduce undue stress on the feet, easing discomfort from prolonged standing or walking.

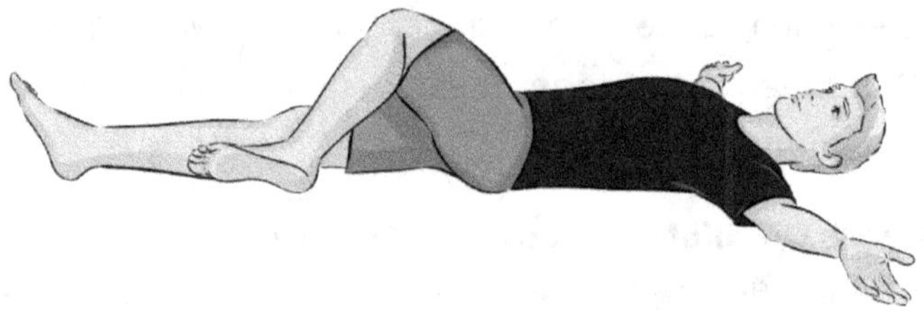

01 **Begin by lying flat on your back on a comfortable surface.** Ensure your spine is in a neutral position.

02 **Extend one leg straight out, while bending the other leg at the knee.** Then, turn the foot and knee inward toward your body. Hold for a second, then release outward back to your knees pointing upward. This triggers pandiculation in outer thigh muscles.

03 Repeat up to 6 times, and do the same with the other leg.

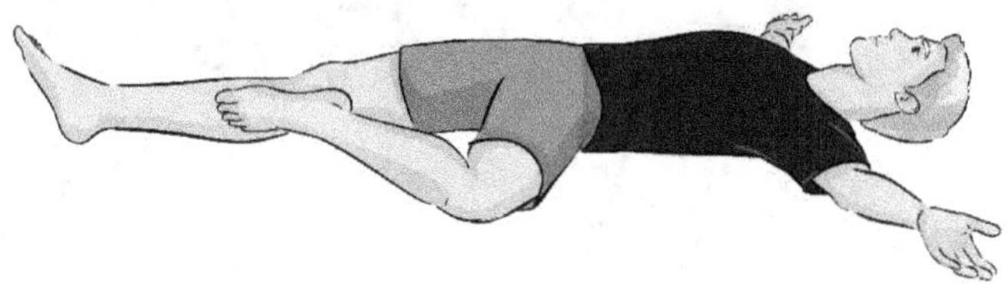

01 **Start by lying flat on your back on a comfortable surface.** Ensure your spine is in a neutral position to minimize strain.

02 **Extend one leg straight out, while bending the other leg at the knee.** Now, turn the foot and knee outward from your body. Hold for a second, then release back to your knees pointing upward. This triggers pandiculation in the inner thigh and adductor muscles.

03 Repeat up to 6 times, and do the same with the other leg.

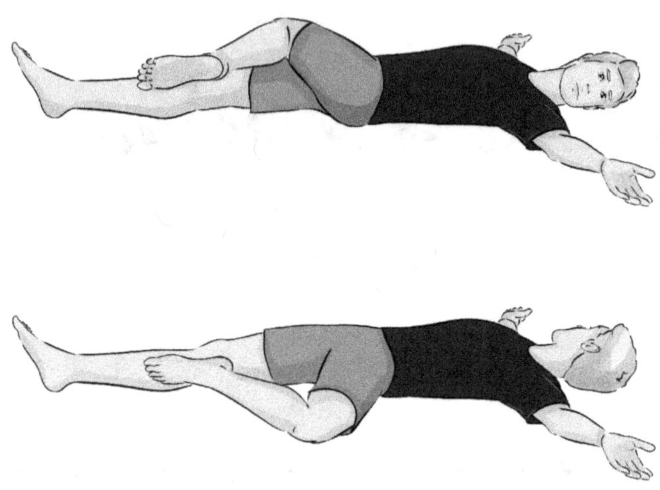

01 **Start by lying flat with your back on a comfortable, flat surface.** Ensure that your spine is aligned and your arms are placed comfortably at your sides. Optional: extend the arms 90 degrees on both sides.

02 **Keep one leg straight along the surface and bend the other leg at the knee.** Now, move the leg with the bent knee inward as your head turns outward. This time, lift your foot off the mat into the air, but keep your foot aligned 90 degrees to your knee as shown in the picture above.

03 Straighten your leg to return to a neutral starting position.

04 **Slowly turn outward. Move your head to the right as your knee moves outward (left). Repeat both movements up to 8 times.**

05 **You should feel a beautiful pandiculation in your neck, arms, and legs.**

06 **After completing the set, relax your foot, leg, and the entire body for a moment.** Notice any changes in the feeling of tension or relaxation in the foot and ankle area.

COMBINATION MOVEMENTS

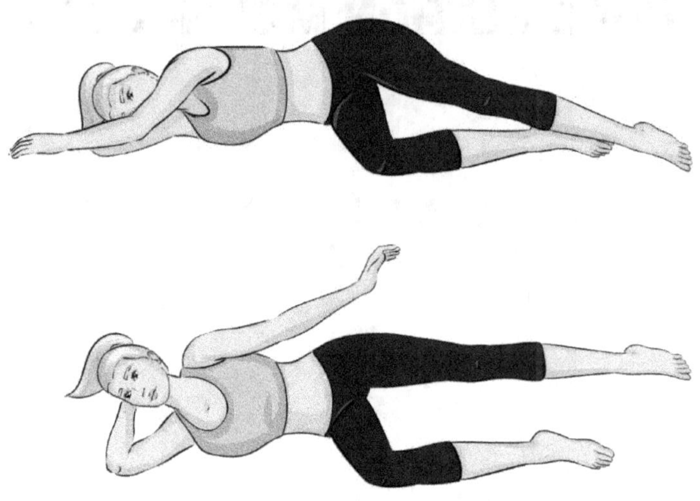

01 The iliotibial (IT) band is a common source of discomfort for many people. Begin by lying on your side on a comfortable surface. Make sure the side of your body experiencing IT band pain is facing upward.

02 Extend the top leg straight in line with the body. Ensure your foot is flexed and your leg is aligned with your torso.

03 Lift the top leg about four inches off the ground. This initial lift engages the muscles along the side of your leg, including the IT band. Your other leg will naturally bend as you do so. Let it.

04 **Place your top hand just above the outside of your thigh, and your other hand holding your head for support.**

Slowly lower your leg back down to the starting position as your hand moves in a counter-clockwise motion down toward the floor by the top of your head. Repeat this movement for up to 4 reps. If done correctly, you will trigger pandiculation on the entire side of your body down to the IT band that's facing up.

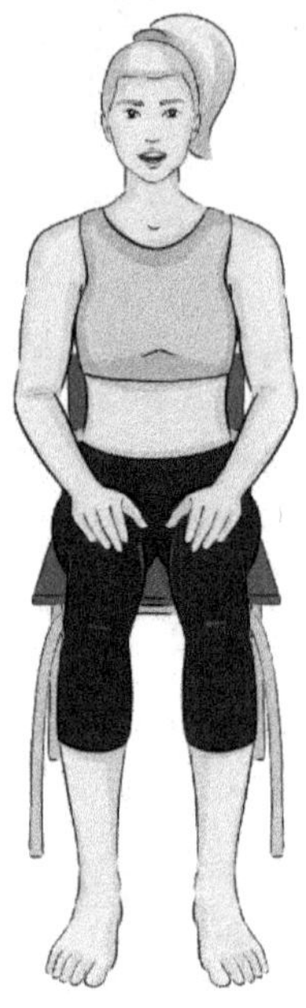 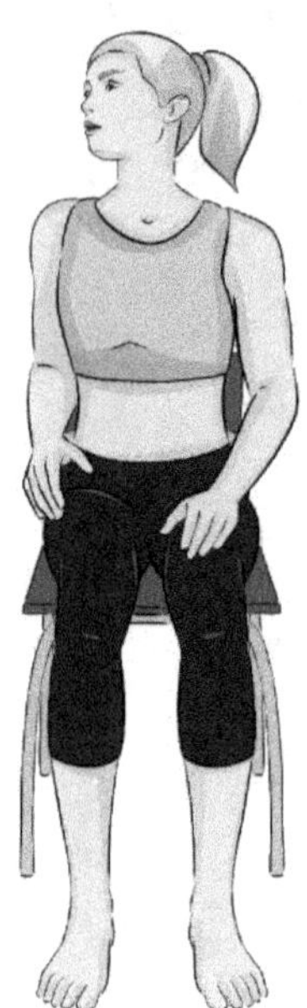

This exercise targets the levator scapula muscle, which runs from the upper cervical vertebrae to the scapula. It helps relieve tension in the neck and shoulder area, commonly caused by poor posture or prolonged sitting.

01   Sit comfortably with your spine straight and shoulders relaxed.

02   Gently turn your head to one side: For stretching the right levator scapula, turn your head to the right. This starts the process of activating the muscle.

03   Introduce a slight side bend towards the same side: Tilt your head so your right ear moves closer to your right shoulder. This increases the stretch in the neck muscle.

04   Bend your elbow on the same side backward and lift your shoulder:
     For the right side, bend your right elbow and lift your right shoulder
     slightly. This helps deepen the stretch by involving the shoulder.
     Hold for 2 seconds.

05   Return to a neutral position. As you do, you will trigger pandiculation
     in your upper neck and trapezius area. Do up to 8 reps.

06   Repeat on the other side.

Developing a Daily Somatic Routine

Developing a daily Somatic routine is about making a personal commitment to become more in tune with the body's language of sensation, which often speaks in whispers before it screams in distress.

Establishing a Foundation

Begin by setting a clear, manageable goal for your daily practice. This might mean dedicating ten minutes each morning to grounding exercises or incorporating mindful stretches at the end of the day. The key is consistency.

Morning Integration

Start your day with grounding. Grounding exercises can be as simple as feeling the floor under your feet, noticing the support of the earth beneath you, or engaging in a full body scan, from the tips of your toes to the top of your head. This practice sets a tone of bodily awareness that carries through the day, helping you remain in the "window of tolerance," where you are best able to cope with stress and remain engaged with your surroundings.

Transition Times

Use transitional moments throughout your day as opportunities to check in with your body. Before and after meetings, while waiting for a meal, or after sending an email, take a moment to notice your breath, posture, and any sensations of discomfort or ease.

Mindful Movement Breaks

Incorporate short, mindful movements into your day to break the cycle of prolonged sitting or standing, which can exacerbate body tension and disconnection. A simple levator release or a yawn into a neck and arm release can easily be done while you are going about your day such as waiting in the office or riding an escalator.

Breathing for Calm

Breath is a powerful tool in regulating the nervous system and can be utilized throughout the day to maintain a calm, centered state. Engage in diaphragmatic breathing, or "belly breathing," to help modulate the stress response and maintain a relaxed state of body and mind. This type of breathing can be particularly effective before stressful events, helping to maintain clarity and presence.

Reflective Practice

End your day with a reflective Somatic practice. This might involve more structured exercises like those found in Somatic experiencing, where you gently explore patterns of tension and relaxation in the body. Alternatively, you might engage in a gentle movement practice or a more formal meditation to reflect on the day, process any lingering stress, and consciously release it.

Integration with Professional Guidance

For those deeply affected by trauma, integrating Somatic practices with professional guidance can enhance the healing journey. Regular sessions with a therapist trained in Somatic experiencing can provide tailored guidance and deeper insights into personal Somatic patterns. These professionals can offer specific exercises that target individual areas of need, helping to accelerate the journey toward Somatic awareness and recovery.

Continual Learning and Adaptation

As you grow in your Somatic practice, continually assess and adapt your routine. What works well today might need adjustment as your body's awareness and needs change. Engage with new learning opportunities, such as workshops or books, and integrate new practices that resonate with your evolving Somatic understanding.

This daily practice is not about rigidly adhering to a set routine but about fostering a living relationship with your body, learning its cues, and responding with kindness and attention.

Troubleshooting Common Challenges in Somatic Exercises

Let's explore the ways to troubleshoot common challenges and adapt these exercises to suit different body types and abilities while addressing issues like discomfort or stagnation in progress.

Adjusting Exercises for Different Body Types and Abilities

1. Recognizing Individual Variability:
Each body carries its unique history; its capabilities and limitations are shaped by personal experiences of joy, injury, illness, and trauma. Somatic exercises should start with acceptance of one's current state, which will differ vastly among individuals.

2. Modification Tips:
For those with limited mobility, begin with exercises that can be performed while seated or lying down, focusing on breath and gentle movements of the arms and head. As confidence and comfort levels improve, gradually introduce movements that extend to the legs and involve mild stretching.

3. Using Props for Support:

Props such as chairs, cushions, yoga mats, and blocks can be invaluable in modifying exercises. For instance, a chair can be used for balance during standing exercises or a cushion can support the back during seated exercises. These tools ensure safety and enhance the effectiveness of the movements.

What to Do If You Experience Discomfort or Lack of Progress

1. Understanding the Source of Discomfort:

Discomfort during exercise can stem from a variety of sources—physical limitations, unresolved trauma surfacing, or simply pushing the body beyond its comfortable range of motion. It is crucial to distinguish between good pain, which is a natural part of muscle growth, and harmful pain, which can signal potential injury or distress.

2. Adjusting Intensity and Duration:

If pain is encountered, reduce the intensity of the movements. Shorten the duration of each exercise session or the individual exercises themselves. It's better to engage briefly but regularly, instead of pushing through pain, which can reinforce trauma responses rather than resolve them.

3. Focusing on Breathing and Relaxation:

Integrate focused breathing techniques to help manage discomfort. Breathing not only oxygenates the muscles and eases tension but also helps ground your mind, making it easier to cope with and interpret bodily sensations.

4. Progress Plateaus:

Lack of progress can be discouraging. It's important to set realistic, incremental goals. Sometimes progress is subtle; it may be beneficial to keep a journal of how you feel before and after each session to track these small changes over time.

5. Seeking Professional Guidance:
If challenges persist, consulting with a professional who understands Somatic practices can provide personalized insights and adjustments. They can offer guidance tailored to your body's needs and help navigate any emotional upheavals that arise during practice.

6. Incorporating Variety and Creativity:
Sometimes, the body becomes accustomed to a certain routine, diminishing the effectiveness of the practice. Introducing new exercises or varying the routine can reengage the body and mind, sparking progress and renewing interest.

7. Community and Shared Experiences:
Joining a group class or community practice can provide support and motivation. Sharing experiences with others can offer new perspectives and strategies for overcoming personal challenges in practice.

Next Steps

"Movement is medicine for creating change in a person's physical, emotional, and mental states."
– Carol Welch

As you integrate these practices into your daily life, their transformative power will gradually manifest, offering increased flexibility, strength, and an enhanced sense of vitality.

After several weeks of consistent practice, these movements will become second nature, part of your daily ritual to maintain and enhance your well-being. For those of you eager to delve deeper into Somatic practices, the journey does not stop here.

I know that some of you will want to continue on more advanced exercises. So, before we say goodbye, let me direct you to our exclusive pelvic floor Kegels exercise guide, at wallpilates.org as taught by Tim Sawyer, a leading physical therapist who worked with Dr. Anderson and Dr. Wise at the Stanford University Medical Center[2]

---

2   Wise, D. & Anderson, R. (2018). *A Headache in the Pelvis: The Wise-Anderson Protocol for Healing Pelvic Pain: The Definitive Edition.*

When you enter your email to download this free bonus, you'll also be notified of new Pilates books and workout routines we release in the future. You can also scan the following QR code to receive your free bonus:

If you have any questions for me, I'll check your emails at wallpilates2@gmail.com.

Wishing you continued success on your wellness journey.

Love,

Luna Light

Use the following URL from the National Pilates Certification Program to find a certified Pilates instructor:

https://nationalpilatescertificationprogram.org/NPCP/NPCP/Directory/CertifiedTeachersList.aspx

Disclosures

Some of the links provided in this book are affiliate links, which will help you jump to the exact URL of the resource you're looking for at no additional cost to you.

References

All stock images from freepiks.com

All illustrations of exercises done in house with full copyright protection.